ALLE ZEIT WACH
1842

H.-M. Hoogewoud

Hepatocellular Carcinoma and Liver Metastases: Diagnosis and Treatment

With a Foreword by A. Rohner

With 41 Figures and 21 Tables

Springer-Verlag
Berlin Heidelberg New York
London Paris Tokyo
Hong Kong Barcelona
Budapest

Henri-Marcel Hoogewoud, MD
Head of the Department of Radiology
Cantonal Hospital
CH-1700 Fribourg, Switzerland

ISBN 3-540-56272-9 Springer-Verlag Berlin Heidelberg New York
ISBN 0-387-56272-9 Springer-Verlag New York Berlin Heidelberg

Library of Congress Cataloging-in-Publication Data. Hoogewoud. H.-M. (Henri-Marcel), 1953– Hepatocellular carcinoma and liver metastases diagnosis and treatment / H.M. Hoogewoud: with a foreword by Adrien Rohner. p. cm. Includes bibliographical references and index. ISBN 3-540-56272-9 (alk. paper)--ISBN 0-387-56272-9 (alk. paper) 1. Liver--Cancer. 2. Liver metastasis. I. Title. [DNLM: 1. Hepatoma--diagnosis. 2. Hepatoma--therapy. 3. Liver Neoplasms--diagnosis. 4. Liver Neoplasms--therapy. 5. Neoplasm Metastasis. WI 735 H779h 1993 RC280.L5H66 1993 616.99′436--dc20 DNLM/DLC for Library of Congress 92-48503

Typesetting: Macmillan India Ltd., Bangalore 25

21/3130/SPS-543210—Printed on acid-free paper

To my wife Danielle and
my daughters Florence and Julie

Foreword

Liver surgery has made extraordinary progress over the past 40 years, evolving from the first, timid partial resections in the 1950s to today's major resections and organ transplants. Examining the reasons for this progress, one cannot but be impressed by the substantial role that has been played by radiology.

Formerly, preoperative planning was based on only nebulous scintigraphic scans. Today, surgeons have at their disposal a wide variety of radiological modalities for diagnosis and topography which are precise enough to exclude most operative surprises. Furthermore, the radiologist is becoming increasingly involved in therapy: *prior to* operation for tumor reduction by embolization and *after* resection for treatment of local complications – which could otherwise necessitate difficult and occasionally dangerous reoperations.

As the author writes in his preface, it is not really astonishing that a radiologist is publishing a book on this topic, and he must be congratulated for his work-up, which combines important personal experience with a complete analysis of published papers on this topic.

Geneva, Switzerland
March 1993

Adrien Rohner

Preface

Liver cancer carries a poor, though not desperate prognosis for survival. Helpful diagnostic and therapeutic modalities exist. The purpose of this book is to provide information about these and to show what can and what should be done when a malignant liver lesion is suspected. I have selected those diagnostic and therapeutic modalities that are currently accepted in the literature in terms of their results and side effects. Anecdotal case reports have been avoided here, except for descriptions of some rare side effects of therapy. Frequent cancer-related conditions are dealt with (hepatocellular carcinoma and metastases), but detailed discussion of tumors with rare histology is beyond the scope of this volume. The literature cited represents a selection of the most important papers published worldwide.

A book on liver cancer written by a radiologist is not common; however, publication of the present volume reflects the increasing role which radiology is now playing in the diagnosis and treatment of cancer. Liver cancer is a perfect example of a field in which a multidisciplinary approach is essential; only teams of surgeons, oncologists, internists, and radiologists working closely together with knowledge and respect for each others' roles are able to be effective. Radiology plays a crucial role in the detection and staging of cancer. Accurate staging assists in selecting patients who may benefit from resection surgery, and can avoid laparotomies being carried out in inoperable patients. Interventional radiology then helps to improve the results of the muldisciplinary therapeutic approach to liver cancer. Embolization and chemoembolization can be of benefit in a selected group of patients, whereas techniques such as abscess drainage are useful in treating complications of therapy. This book should provide the reader with useful information about the possibilities of modern radiology.

Fribourg, Switzerland
March 1993

Henri-Marcel Hoogewoud

Acknowledgments

I am grateful to the many people who have helped in realizing this book. First, I want to thank Dr. Paul Pugin, oncologist at the Cantonal Hospital of Fribourg, with whom I have shared hopes and fears in the diagnosis and treatment of liver cancer patients. I thank him for his help in revising the manuscript, for his suggestions, and for his support. His constant presence and his devotion are a great support for patients and for the medical staff. I am grateful to the surgeons of our hospital for their help. My thanks also go to Prof. Adrien Rohner, head of the Department of Surgery at the University Hospital of Geneva for honoring this publication with a foreword. I wish to thank Dr. Rudolf Steffen, a well-known liver surgeon with very extensive experience in the field of resection surgery and transplantation for reviewing the surgical part of the manuscript. I am very grateful to Prof. François Terrier, head of the Department of Radiology at the University Hospital of Geneva, and to Prof. Reinhard Kraft, Institute of Pathology, University of Bern, for reviewing the manuscript and for their suggestions. I wish to express my gratitude to the radiologists and the technicians of my Department for their help and support. Finally, I thank M. Arthur J. Grainger for all the photographic work that he has done for me.

Fribourg, Switzerland
March 1993

H.-M. Hoogewoud

Contents

1 Anatomy of the Liver 1

1.1 Hepatic Veins 2
1.2 Portal Vein 4
1.3 Hepatic Arteries 5
1.4 Biliary Ducts 5
1.5 Lymphatic Drainage 5

2 Malignant Liver Lesions: Pathology 9

2.1 Hepatocellular Carcinoma 9
2.1.1 Epidemiology 9
2.1.2 Pathology 11
2.2 Hepatoblastoma 14
2.3 Cholangiocarcinoma 14
2.4 Mesenchymal Tumors 14
2.4.1 Angiosarcoma (Hemangioendothelioma) 14
2.4.2 Other Mesenchymal Tumors 15
2.5 Metastases 15

3 Diagnosis and Staging of Malignant Liver Disease 18

3.1 Clinical Aspects 18
3.1.1 Hepatocellular Carcinomas 18
3.1.2 Metastases 19
3.2 Biochemical Tests 19
3.3 Techniques in Imaging Malignant Liver Disease . . 20
3.3.1 Plain Film 20
3.3.2 Ultrasound 21
3.3.3 Computed Tomography 23
3.3.4 Magnetic Resonance 27
3.3.5 Angiography 28
3.3.6 Nuclear Medicine 30
3.4 Imaging Malignant Focal Liver Lesions 31
3.4.1 Hepatocellular Carcinoma 31

3.4.2 Liver Metastases 32
3.4.3 Cholangiocarcinoma 33
3.4.4 Lymphoma 34
3.4.5 Fatty Infiltration 34
3.5 Percutaneous Liver Biopsy 34
3.5.1 Biopsy of Malignant Liver Lesions 35
3.5.2 Biopsy of Liver Hemangiomas 38
3.5.3 Complications of Biopsy 38
3.6 Principles of Staging of Liver Lesions 39
3.7 Which Method to Choose? 40

4 Surgical Treatment of Malignant Liver Lesions 44

4.1 Liver Resection 44
4.1.1 Criteria for Resection 44
4.1.2 Tumorectomy 47
4.1.3 Segmentectomy and Hepatectomy 48
4.1.4 Results and Factors Influencing Survival 48
4.1.5 Complications of Resection Surgery 54
4.2 Arterial Ligature: Dearterialization 55
4.2.1 Techniques 56
4.2.2 Results 56
4.3 Cryosurgery 57
4.4 Transplantation 58

5 Radiotherapy 62

5.1 Tolerance of the Liver to Radiation 62
5.2 External Radiotherapy 62
5.2.1 Irradiation with Curative Intention 63
5.2.2 Irradiation with Palliative Intention 63
5.2.3 Tolerance to Treatment and Complications 64
5.3 Internal Radiotherapy 64
5.3.1 Percutaneous Implantation of Radioactive Seeds .. 64
5.3.2 Yttrium-90 64
5.3.3 ^{131}I-Labeled Lipiodol 65
5.3.4 Radiolabeled Antibodies 65
5.4 Radiotherapy Combined with Chemotherapy 67

6 Ethanol Injection Therapy of Liver Tumors 70

6.1 Patient Selection 70
6.2 Technique 70
6.3 Results 72

7 Systemic Chemotherapy 74

7.1 Tumor Response to Chemotherapy 74
7.2 Hepatocellular Carcinomas 74
7.3 Liver Metastases 76

8 Selective Perfusion of Chemotherapeutic Agents 79

8.1 General Considerations 79
8.1.1 Regional Chemotherapy: High Local Concentration of Drugs 79
8.1.2 Anatomic Considerations: Vascular Remodeling . . 81
8.1.3 Flow Pattern: Laminar Flow–Turbulent Flow 83
8.1.4 Checking the Homogeneity of Liver Perfusion . . . 84
8.2 Regional Chemotherapy: The “Surgical Way” 84
8.2.1 Intraarterial Regional Chemotherapy 85
8.2.2 Portal Versus Intraarterial Chemotherapy 86
8.2.3 Adjuvant Intraportal Chemotherapy for Colorectal Hepatic Metastases 86
8.2.4 Adjuvant Intraperitoneal Chemotherapy for Colorectal Hepatic Metastases 87
8.3 Regional Chemotherapy: the “Radiological” Way . 88
8.3.1 Intraarterial Perfusion 89
8.3.2 Chemotherapeutic Drugs and Lipiodol 90
8.3.3 Embolization 91
8.3.4 Chemoembolization 93
8.4 Complications and Side Effects of Regional Chemotherapy 101

Subject Index 109

1 Anatomy of the Liver

Knowledge of the anatomy and segmental nature of the liver is essential in the management of patients with malignant liver lesions. Precise localization of the lesions is important as the feasibility and the type of a surgical treatment depend on it. The identification of anatomical landmarks in the liver with imaging modalities such as ultrasound, computed tomography (CT), and magnetic resonance (MR) allows precise localizing of liver lesions.

The liver weighs about 1500 g and is divided into two lobes and eight segments (Fig. 1.1). The division of the liver is based on vascular territories that produce potential surgical intersegmental and interlobar planes containing the hepatic veins [1,2]. The landmarks and the vessels delimiting the segments can be recognized with imaging techniques and help to localize lesions in the liver parenchyma (Figs. 1.2–1.4).

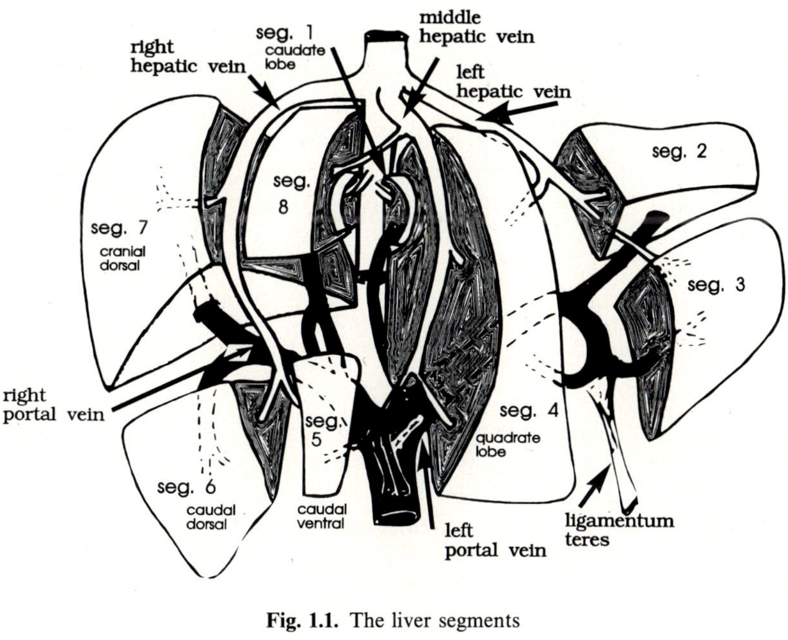

Fig. 1.1. The liver segments

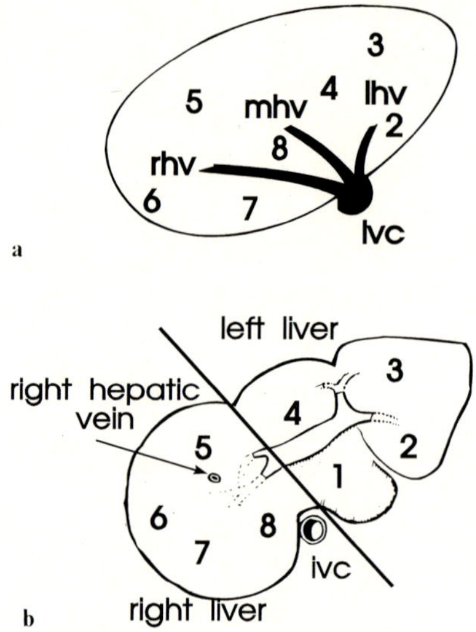

Fig. 1.2. **a** The liver segments, oblique. *lhv*, Left hepatic vein; *mhv*, middle hepatic vein; *rhv*, right hepatic vein. **b** The liver segments; the liver is seen from below

The plane between the inferior vena cava and the main middle hepatic vein separates the right from the left lobe. The left lobe is separated into two portions by the portoumbilical fissure formed by the falciform ligament containing caudally the obliterated umbilical vein (ligamentum teres hepatis), venous ligament (Arantii), and hepatogastric ligament. At the cranial diaphragmatic aspect of the liver, the falciform ligament separates into right and left coronary ligaments that define the extraperitoneal bare area of the liver. On both sides the coronary ligaments end up in the triangular ligaments. The porta hepatis contains the portal vein dorsally and the hepatic artery with the vegetative nervous tissue, extrahepatic biliary tract, and portal lymphatics ventrally.

About 75% of the blood supply to the liver is obtained through the portal veins and the remaining 25% through the hepatic arteries.

1.1 Hepatic Veins

Although there is considerable variation, the hepatic venous drainage consists generally of left, middle, and right hepatic veins.

The middle hepatic vein drains most of the blood from segment 4 (the quadrate lobe) of the left lobe and from segments 5 and 8 from the right lobe. The left hepatic vein lies in a plane separating segment 4, located medially, from segments 2 and 3 located laterally in the left lobe. As the left hepatic vein separates early into smaller branches, it can be identified only in the cranial

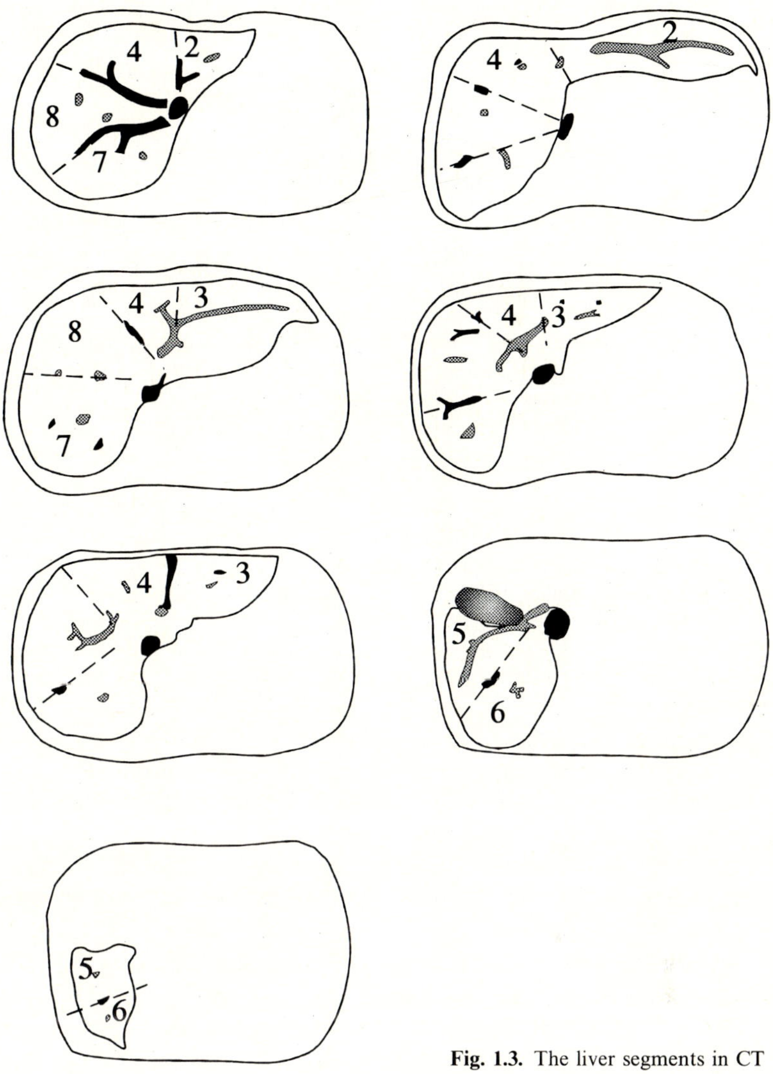

Fig. 1.3. The liver segments in CT

aspect of the separation plane. The caudal aspect of this plane is delimited by the ligamentum teres, umbilical fissure, and falciform ligament. In the right lobe, the right hepatic vein separates the dorsal segments 6 and 7 from the anterior segments 5 and 8. The right hepatic vein drains segments 6 and 7 and the dorsal aspect of the ventral segments 5 and 8.

The caudate lobe (segment 1) must be considered as a separate entity. It lies left and anterior to the inferior vena cava. It is drained independently by one or more veins entering the inferior vena cava directly.

The three main veins enter the inferior vena cava in the high subdiaphragmatic portion of the liver. The left and the middle hepatic veins may form

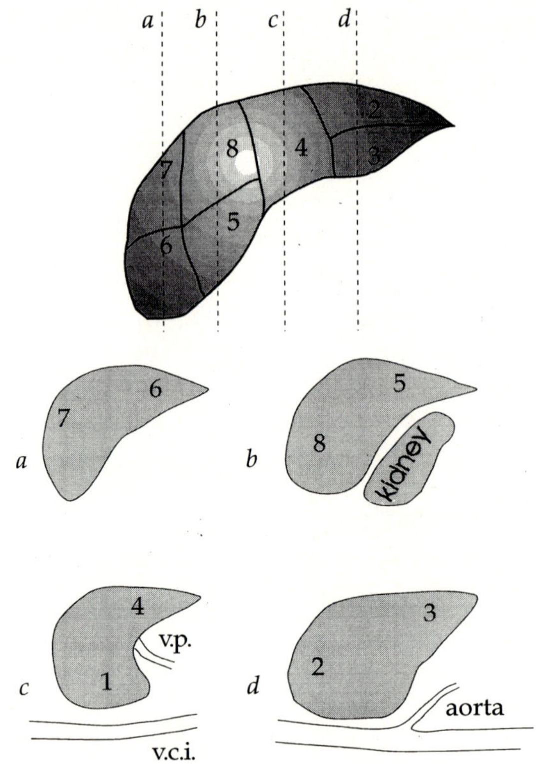

Fig. 1.4. The liver segments in ultrasound, seen along the sagittal plane

a common trunk or enter the inferior vena cava separately. The right hepatic vein usually enters separately. There are numerous other small hepatic veins draining the liver independently, but these are usually too small to be recognized on CT or ultrasound.

1.2 Portal Vein

The portal vein carries splanchnic blood to the liver and is formed by the confluence of the superior mesenteric, splenic, and inferior mesenteric veins. It is about 8 cm long, courses cephalad and rightward and divides into right and left portal veins. The right portal vein varies from 0 to 3 cm in length, lies anterior to the caudate lobe, and divides soon into anterior and posterior branches. The anterior branch divides into ascending branches (to segment 8) and descending branches (to segment 5). The posterior branch also divides into ascending branches (to segment 7) and descending branches (to segment 6). The left portal vein, about 4 cm long, lies anterior to the caudate lobe and courses leftward to reach the portoumbilical fissure where it enters the liver substance. At this point it is joined anteriorly by the round ligament (ligamentum teres hepatis). Two branches arise laterally to join segments 2 and 3. After a sharp curve the left portal vein enters the quadrate lobe (segment 4) from the right side and divides into ascending and descending branches.

The caudate lobe is supplied from one or more branches arising from the portal bifurcation or from the right or left portal vein.

1.3 Hepatic Arteries

The arterial supply of the liver is subject to considerable variation (Figs. 1.5, 1.6), commonly noted variations being a right hepatic branch from the superior mesenteric artery and a left hepatic branch from the left gastric artery. The hepatic artery divides into right and left main branches. The location of the division is inconstant. The caudate lobe receives blood from small branches arising from the right and left hepatic arteries.

1.4 Biliary Ducts

The anatomy of the biliary ducts reflect the anatomy of the portal veins. The biliary ducts are enclosed with the portal veins and the hepatic arteries in a connective sheath (Glisson). On the right side the segments 7 and 6 are drained by posterior ascending and descending branches and the segments 8 and 5 by anterior ascending and descending branches. On the left side two lateral branches drain the lateral segments 2 and 3, and one medial branch drains segment 4. The caudate lobe drains separately into the right and left hepatic ducts.

1.5 Lymphatic Drainage

The lymph of the liver drains into a superficial and a deep system [3]. The superficial lymphatic vessels, located in the subserous tissue, drain in four directions: (a) The middle part of the posterior surface, caudate lobe, posterior part of the inferior surface of the right lobe, and posterior part of the convex surfaces of both lobes drain into vessels to nodes around the terminal part of the inferior vena cava. Vessels located in the coronary and right triangular ligaments may drain directly into the thoracic duct. (b) The lymphatic vessels

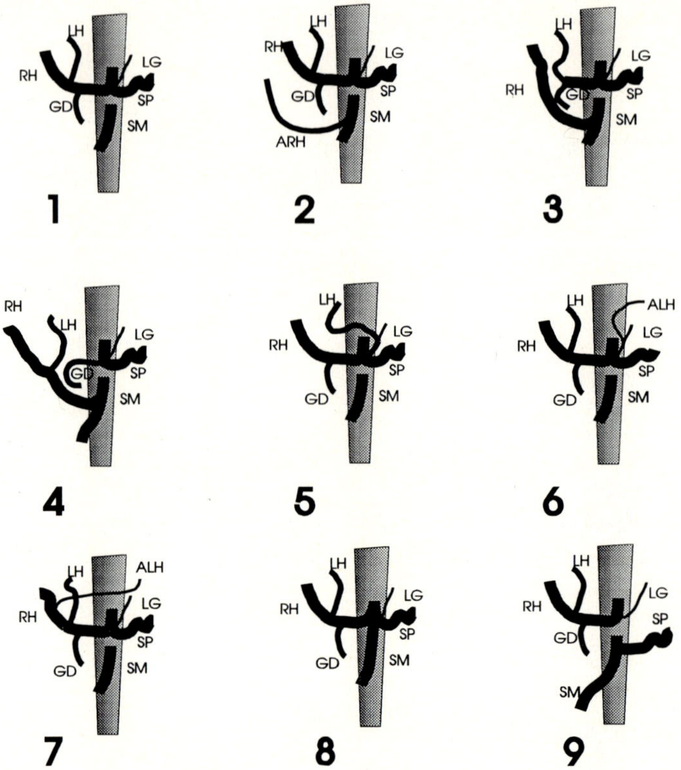

Fig. 1.5. Frequently found variations in the vascular supply of the liver. *ALH*, Accessory left hepatic artery; *ARH*, accessory right hepatic artery; *GD*, gastroduodenal artery; *LG*, left gastric artery; *LH*, left hepatic artery; *RH*, right hepatic artery; *SM*, superior mesenteric artery; *SP*, splenic artery. *1*, Normal anatomy; *2*, accessory right hepatic artery from superior mesenteric; *3*, right hepatic artery from superior mesenteric artery; *4*, common hepatic artery from superior mesenteric artery; *5*, left hepatic from left gastric; *6*, acessory left hepatic from left gastric, *7*, accessory left hepatic from right hepatic; *8*, superior mesenteric artery from celiac trunc; *9*, splenic artery from superior mesenteric artery

of the anterior parts of the inferior surface and of the convex surface near the attachment of the falciform ligament converge to the porta hepatis to drain into the hepatic nodes. (c) Parts of the left lobe are drained by vessels passing through the esophageal hiatus and ending in the paracardial nodes. (d) One or two lymphatic trunks drain the remaining convex surface of the right lobe and follow the inferior phrenic artery across the right diaphragmatic crus to the celiac nodes. The deep hepatic lymphatic system drains into an ascending trunk following the hepatic veins and ending in the nodes round the end of the inferior vena cava and into a descending trunk following the porta hepatis ending in the hepatic nodes.

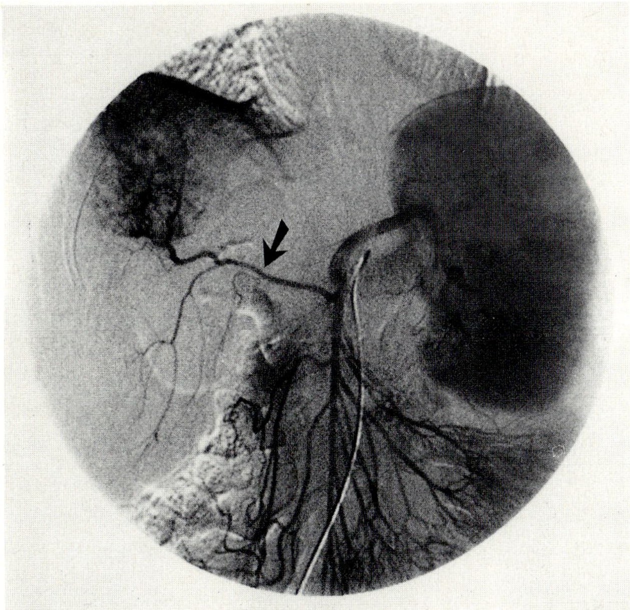

a

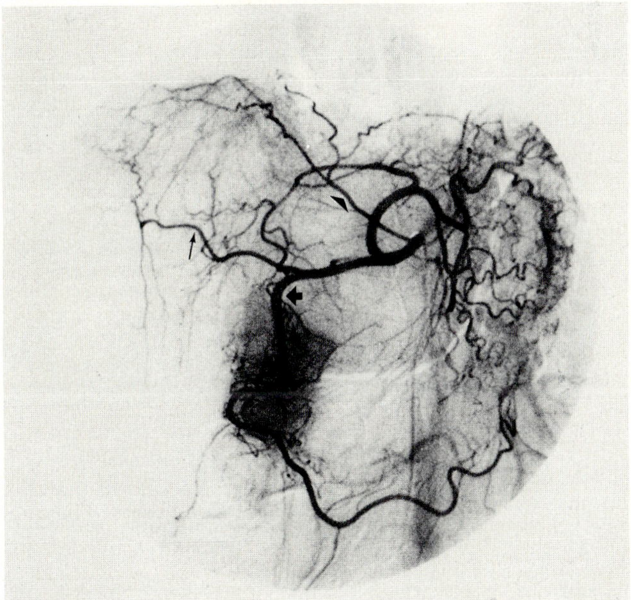

b

Fig. 1.6. **a** Right hepatic artery (*arrow*) feeding a tumor and splenic artery originate in superior mesenteric artery. **b** Accessory right hepatic (*sharp little arrow*) and left hepatic artery, the gastroduodenal (*black arrow*), the phrenic (*arrowhead*), and the left gastric artery originate directly from the aorta

References

1. Couinaud C (1957) Le foie: études anatomiques et chirurgicales. Masson, Paris, pp 9–12
2. Bismuth H (1982) Surgical anatomy and anatomical surgery of the liver. World J Surg 6: 3–9
3. Warwick R, Williams PL (eds) (1973) Gray's anatomy. Longman, Harlow

2 Malignant Liver Lesions: Pathology

The liver is one of the favorite sites for metastatic cancer, providing a suitable environment for the growth of neoplastic cells. Malignant lymphomas, leukemic cells, metastases and primary liver tumors develop readily within this organ. The dual blood supply, size of the organ, and abundant availability of nutritional material are factors favoring tumor growth [1].

Primary liver neoplasms may arise from hepatocytes, biliary epithelium, or mesenchymal structures. Benign tumors include liver cell adenomas, bile duct adenomas, cavernous hemangiomas, and hemangioendotheliomas of infancy. Malignant tumors comprise hepatocellular carcinomas, carcinomas arising from the biliary tract, mesenchymal tumors, and metastatic tumors. Most liver carcinomas derive from the hepatic cells; about 15%–25% arise from bile duct cells.

2.1 Hepatocellular Carcinoma

2.1.1 Epidemiology

Primary liver carcinoma holds a special position among malignant neoplasms as it often arises in an organ that is already severely damaged by cirrhosis. Worldwide, the frequency of liver cell carcinomas varies by as much as 100-fold. Liver cell carcinomas are found in 0.1%–0.7% of all autopsies in Europe and in the United States. In regions with low incidence, between 4% and 6% of patients with cirrhosis develop carcinoma of the liver, which contrasts with some areas in Africa where the frequency is about 40% of all persons with cirrhosis. Although the etiology of liver cell carcinomas is not established, it is known that hepatitis B and aflatoxins are often involved.

Relation to Hepatitis

A high familiar incidence of HBsAg positive liver cell carcinomas has been found in families in Japan. Family members without liver carcinoma were shown to have chronic active viral hepatitis B, chronic persistent viral hepatitis B, or inactive viral cirrhosis B [2]. There is a strong relationship between the rate of

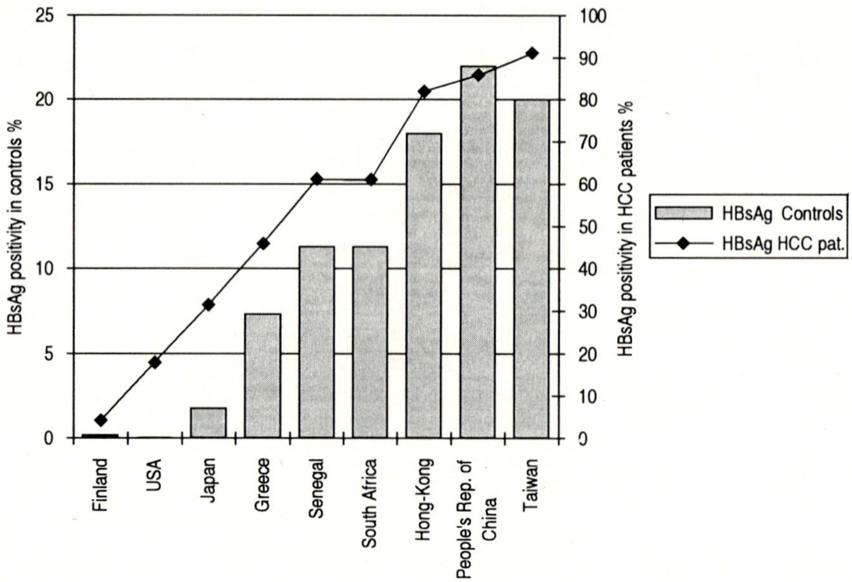

Fig. 2.1. Rates of HBsAG positivity in the population and in patients with hepatocellular carcinoma in various countries (compiled from [12])

HBsAg and the rate of hepatocellular carcinoma in a given population; both are high in sub-Saharian Africa and the Far East and low in the United States and Northern Europe (see Fig. 2.1). A chart of global distribution of prevalence levels of hepatitis B infection is shown in Fig. 2.2.

There is recent evidence of association between hepatocellular carcinoma and non-A and non-B hepatitis; cases after posttransfusion non-A, non-B hepatitis have been reported [3]. Chronic hepatitis C virus infection seems also to play an important role in the pathogenesis of hepatocellular carcinoma, especially in patients with cirrhosis unrelated to alcohol or hepatitis B virus infection [4].

Toxins

It is now established that aflatoxin, a metabolite of the fungus *Aspergillus flavus*, plays an important role in the etiology of hepatocellular carcinoma. *A. flavus* is widespread in humid parts of the world where it grows on peanuts, soybeans, and cereals. Aflatoxin B_1 is the most toxic of the aflatoxins and is highly carcinogenic to some species. Countries such as Mozambique, Transkei, Swaziland, and Kenya with a high daily intake of aflatoxin have a high frequency of liver cell carcinomas [5, 6] (see Fig. 2.3).

Alkaloids from a variety of plants, dietary factors such as cycasin from cycad nuts in endemic areas in Asia, Africa, and South America, and nitrosamines are

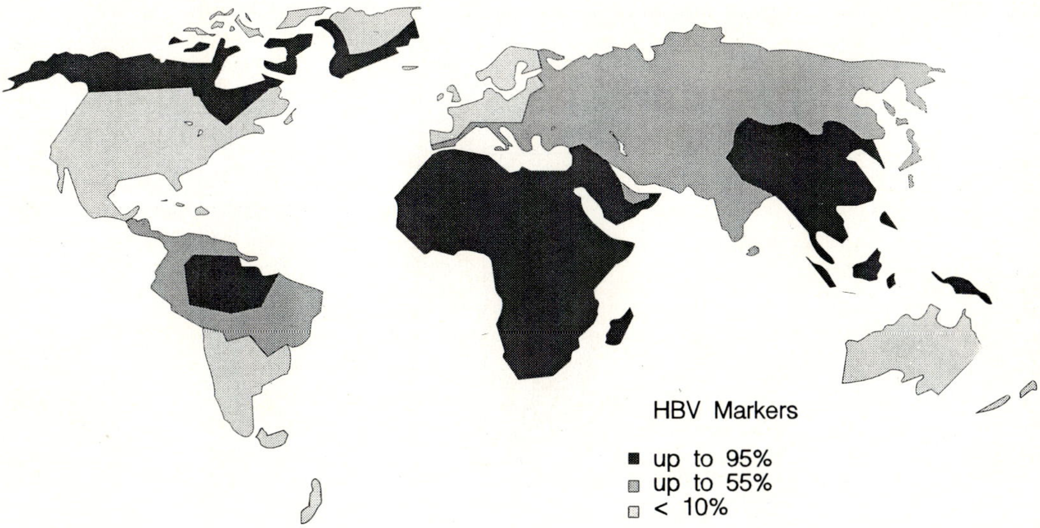

Fig. 2.2. Global distribution of prevalance levels of hepatitis B infection. Adapted from WHO EPI Update November 1989

also carcinogenic [7]. High doses of iron in beer made in iron receptacles has also been implicated as a causative factor of hepatocellular carcinoma in African Bantu populations. Tobacco smoking is a dose-dependent risk factor for hepatocellular carcinoma in hepatitis B surface antigen (HBsAg) negative patients [8].

Cirrhosis

How cirrhosis predisposes to liver cell carcinoma is not clearly understood. Precancerous changes, however, in the form of large atypical cells containing hyperchromatic polyploid nuclei and binucleate forms, are often found in advanced cirrhosis, especially when large regenerative nodules are present. A possible explanation is that synthesis of DNA is accelerated in regenerative nodules, and thus rearrangements of DNA sequences may occur more frequently. Livers with micronodular cirrhosis, as found in alcoholic patients, have less regenerative activity. This activity increases during abstinence, small regenerative nodules being transformed into large ones. Hepatocellular carcinomas seem to appear rarely in patients with alcoholic liver disease while they are drinking. In Western countries the alcoholic micronodular type of cirrhosis is more frequently encountered than in the Far East where the posthepatitic type predominates.

2.1.2 Pathology

Liver cell carcinomas are either massive, nodular, or diffuse and arise mostly in livers with advanced cirrhosis. The α-fetoprotein level is frequently elevated

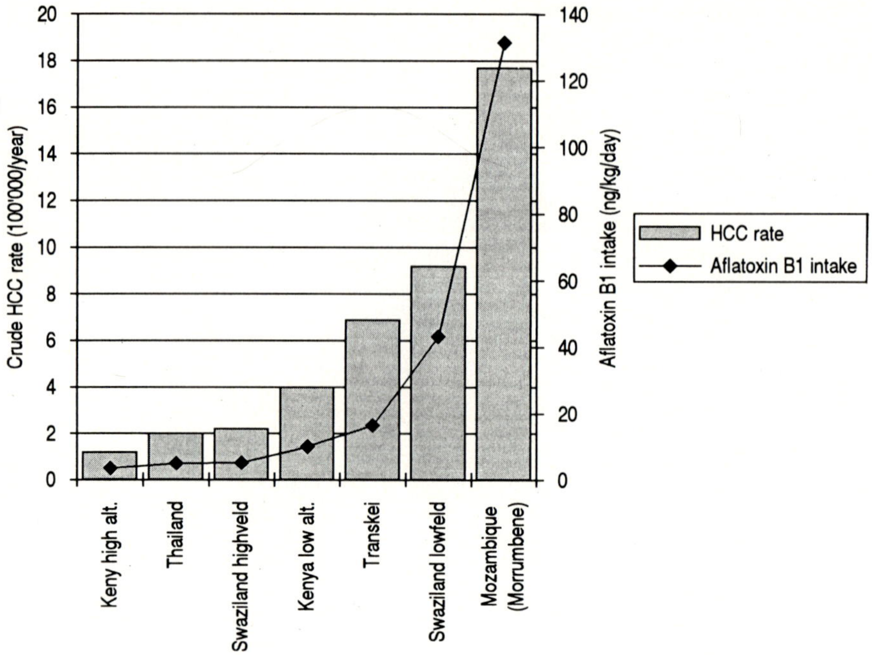

Fig. 2.3. Relation of aflatoxin intake and crude hepatocellular carcinoma rate [24]

(>100 ng/ml). The liver is generally enlarged, the right lobe being most often involved in the massive and nodular forms of the carcinoma. Tumor nodules may bulge below the liver capsule and are softer than regenerative nodules of the cirrhotic liver. In the nodular type, one nodule is generally bigger than the others and may be considered as the primary lesion. Hemorrhage and necrosis are frequent in tumor nodules. Invasion of the portal trunk and/or branches of the portal vein, which was encountered in about 65% of 232 autopsy cases of hepatocellular carcinoma [9], is probably responsible for tumor spread throughout the whole organ. Growth in larger portal branches may induce thrombosis of the portal trunk and secondarily portal hypertension. Invasion of hepatic veins is common; this explains why the lung is the organ in which metastases are found most frequently. A tumor thrombus may extend into the inferior vena cava and allow the spreading of the tumor in to the lungs and more distant locations. Invasion of bile ducts is found in about 9.2% of cases [10] and may mimic gallstone disease in clinical presentation.

In the massive form, the tumor, generally located in the right liver lobe, consists of a solid mass that may be accompanied by one or several satellite nodules. The diffuse type consists of small nodules that are sometimes hard to differentiate from cirrhosis. Hepatocellular carcinoma cells often retain morphological characteristics of normal liver cells with large hyperchromatic nuclei

Table 2.1. Metastatic spread of hepatocellular carcinoma (data compiled from [13])

Location	Frequency(%)
Hematogenous metastases	
Lung	51.6
Adrenal	8.4
Bone	5.8
Meninges	5.4
Pancreas	3.1
Brain	2.7
Kidney	2.2
Lymphogenous metastases	
Hepatic hilum	14.1
Head of pancreas	10.7
Aorta	7.0
Retroperitoneum	5.8
Stomach	5.3
Mediastinum	4.9
Trachea	4.9
Carina	4.0
Neck	3.1
Virschow node	2.2
Direct infiltration or dissemination	
Diaphragm	10.2
Douglas	6.2
Gallblader	5.8
Peritoneal dissemination	4.0

and abundant granular cytoplasm. Trabecular growth as well as many functions of normal liver cells such as bile, fat, or glycogen production are found. Intense sclerosis around neoplastic tubular structures characterizes the sclerosing hepatocellular carcinoma variant.

The fibrolamellar variant is a form of hepatocellular carcinoma found in adolescents and young adults. No predisposing risk factors are known at present, and the patients do not have an underlying cirrhosis. The α-fetoprotein level is normal. Growing as a solid mass, the tumor may have satellite nodules. Radiologically it may be confused with focal nodular hyperplasia because of its central fibrous scar. The mass may be totally or partially encapsulated. Polygonal, eosinophilic hepatocytes are embedded in abundant fibrous stroma. Prognosis is better than for conventional hepatocellular carcinoma as resectability and 5-year survival after resection are higher.

Metastases of hepatocellular carcinomas have been found everywhere (Table 2.1), but especially in lungs. Metastases have been found in varices, even if sclerosed [11, 12], representing a potential route for lung metastases. Locoregional lymph nodes in the porta hepatis are often involved.

2.2 Hepatoblastoma

Hepatoblastoma is a rare tumor occurring in infancy and early childhood in both sexes. It presents as progressive enlargement of the abdomen, fever, rarely jaundice, anorexia, and failure to thrive. Hepatoblastoma is sometimes associated with sexual precocity (due to ectopic secretion of gonadotrophin by the tumor), renal adenomas, hemiatrophy, and cystathioninuria. The serum levels of α-fetoprotein are markedly increased. Histologically, the tumor displays a recapitulation of the development stages of the liver. Generally the cells are arranged in acini, pseudorosettes, or papillary formation and are of fetal or embryonic type. Since the tumor usually presents as a solitary mass, it is more often resectable than hepatocellular carcinoma and is associated with a higher 5-year survival rate.

2.3 Cholangiocarcinoma

Cholangiocarcinomas are tumors arising from the biliary ducts. No evident association with hepatitis B or cirrhosis has been proven. An increased incidence is found in patients presenting a chronic biliary obstruction and infection, such as in sclerosing cholangitis, inflammatory bowel disease, and Caroli's disease. Etiologic factors of cholangiocarcinoma include *Clonorchis sinensis* infestation, fibrocystic disease, anabolic steroids, and thorotrast (colloidal solution of α-ray emitting thorium dioxide used formerly as a contrast medium in radiology) [14]. Generally cholangiocarcinomas arise in larger bile ducts involving in at least one third of cases the intrahepatic ducts and the proximal parts of common bile duct. Cholangiocarcinomas arise in 10%–26% of the instances at the confluence of the hepatic ducts (Klatskin tumors [15]) [16]. Simultaneous occurrence with hepatocellular carcinoma has been described [17]. Cholangiocarcinomas are usually mucin-producing, well-differentiated, sclerosing adenocarcinomas that can be difficult to distinguish from metastatic adenocarcinomas. The tumor cells sometimes have a papillary or a tubular arrangement simulating bile ducts. Some cholangiocarcinomas are of the squamous cell type. The prognosis is poor; only 5% of patients survive 5 years [18]. Death is often caused by the complications of biliary obstruction: cholangitis, liver abscesses, biliary cirrhosis, and portal hypertension.

2.4 Mesenchymal Tumors

2.4.1 Angiosarcoma (Hemangioendothelioma)

This rare and highly malignant tumor occurs in older age groups and is difficult to distinguish from hepatocellular carcinoma. Etiological factors in

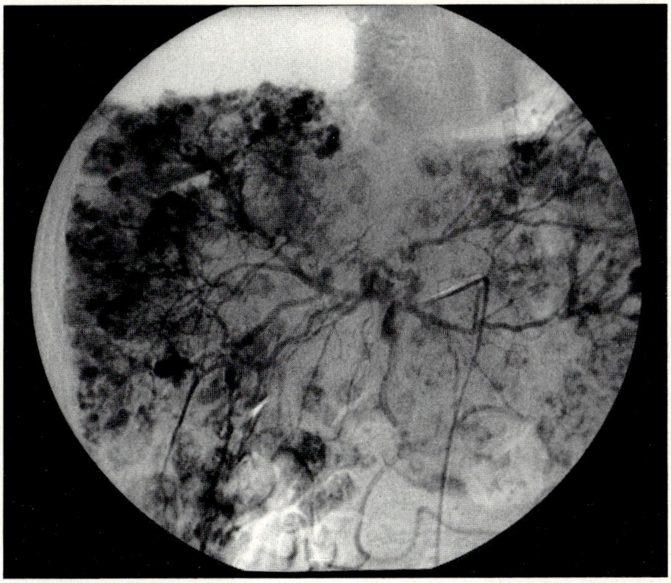

Fig. 2.4. Angiograph of an angiosarcoma. The angiograph rather than a picture of the biopsy was chosen to show the extreme hypervascularity of this diffusely infiltrative tumor in a 45 years old painter having a long history of working with solvents

hemangioendothelioma include thorotrast, vinyl chloride, arsenic, and androgenic-anabolic steriods [19]. Blood-filled sinuses lined with undifferentiated, anaplastic endothelial cells are found histologically. The cells resemble the earliest stages of embryonic vascular development. Spread into the portal venous and the hepatic venous system is frequently encountered. The prognosis is very poor. The tumor is considered to be nonradiosensitive. An example of angiosarcoma is shown in Fig. 2.4.

2.4.2 Other Mesenchymal Tumors

Other mesenchymal elements of the liver have been identified as precursors to malignant tumors. Sarcomatous neoplasias such as mixed hepatic tumors, malignant mesenchymomas and embryonal rhabdomyosarcoma are rare and occur specially in infancy and childhood. A few cases of fibrosarcoma [20] and leiomyosarcoma have been described.

2.5 Metastases

About 40%–50% of neoplasms show liver metastases at death. The most frequently involved cancers are those drained by the portal system, breast, lung, and malignant melanoma. Tumors drained by the portal vein account for 48% of the tumors metastatic to the liver [21]. The presentation of liver metastases may vary from a microscopic solitary nodule to an enormous liver weighing several kilograms and full of bulky masses. The center of metastatic nodules is often soft, necrotic, or hemorrhagic as the metastases may have outgrown their blood supply. Invasion of portal radicles or perivascular lymphatics contributes, by direct spread, to a further metastatization in the liver. Presence of ascites reflects peritoneal involvement or sometimes thrombosis in the portal venous system. Deep jaundice may be caused by invasion of major bile ducts.

The liver is a common site for secondary spread. This cannot be explained merely by the fact that portal venous drainage carries tumor emboli from the gastrointestinal tumors, as cancers from extraportal sites commonly metastasize to the liver. Filtering of circulating cancer cells by target organs does not necessarily mean induction of metastases, as most cells are killed within 24 h. This relative "metastatic inefficiency" of circulating cancer cells has been confirmed in several animal models. As opposed to this passive model of cells being filtered in certain organs, more active processes should be considered in metastatic spread. Specific cell binding patterns [22] or individual responses to organ growth factors [23] probably explain why certain cancer cells prefer special target organs for metastatic spread (organotropism). Various populations of cells with different behavior can coexist in a cancer. Some have a high metastatic potential and may outgrow their nonmetastatic counterparts. During growth, the metastatic potential of a primary tumor may vary, and subpopulations of cells can show a predilection for certain metastatic sites. Knowing that cancer cells can vary their behavior during growth and express various degrees of malignancy may be important for developing new therapeutic modalities, which ultimately will influence patient survival.

References

1. Kemeny N, Schneider A (1989) Regional treatment of hepatic metastastases and hepatocellular carcinoma. Curr Probl Cancer 13(4): 197–283
2. Ohbayashi A (1976) Genetic and familial aspects of liver cirrhosis and hepatocellular carcinoma. In: Okuda K, Peters RL (eds) Hepatocellular carcinoma. Wiley, New York
3. Resnick RH, Stone K, Antonioli D (1983) Primary hepatocellular carcinoma following non-A, non-B post-transfusion hepatitis. Dig Dis Sci 28: 908–911
4. Zala C, Havelka, J, Althofer J, Joller-Jemelka HJ, Risti B, Meier B, Schmid M, Bühler H (1992) Hepatitis-C-Virus und Hepatom. Schweiz Med Wochenschr 122: 194–197
5. Peers FG, Linsell CA (1973) Dietary aflatoxins and liver cell cancer – a population based study in Kenya. Br J Cancer 27: 473–484
6. Linsell CA, Peers FG (1977) Aflatoxin and liver cell cancer. Trans R Soc Trop Med Hyg 71: 471–473
7. Farber E (1984) Pre-cancerous steps in carcinogenesis : their physiological adaptive nature. Biochim Biophys Acta 738: 171
8. Trichopoulos D, Day NE, Kaklamani E, Tzonou A, Munoz N, Zavitsanos X, Koumantaki Y, Trichopoulou A (1987) Hepatitis B virus, tobacco smoking and ethanol consumption in etiology of hepatocellular carcinoma. Int J Cancer 39: 45–49

9. Nakashima T, Okuda K, Kojiro M et al. (1983) Pathology of hepatocellular carcinoma in Japan. 232 consecutive cases autopsied in ten years. Cancer 51: 863–877
10. Kojiro M, Kawabata K, Kawano Y, Shirai F, Takemoto N, Nakashima T (1982) Hepatocellular carcinoma presenting as intrabile duct tumor growth: a clinicopathologic study of 24 cases. Cancer 49: 2144–2147
11. Hiraoka T, Iwai K, Yamashita R, Tada I, Miyauchi Y (1986) Metastases from hepatocellular carcinoma in sclerosed oesophageal varices in cirrhotic patients. Br J Surg 73: 932
12. Arakawa M, Kage M, Matsumoto S, Akagi Y, Noda T, Fukuda K, Nakashima T, Okuda K (1986) Frequency and significance of tumor thrombi in oesophageal varices in hepatocellular carcinoma associated with cirrhosis. Hepatology 6: 419–422
13. Okuda K, Okuda H (1991) Primary liver cell carcinoma. In: McIntyre N, Benhamou JP, Bircher J, Rizetto M, Rodes J (eds) Oxford textbook of clinical hepatology. Oxford University Press, Oxford
14. Goodman ZD, Ishak KG, Langloss JM, Sesterhenn IA, Rabin L (1985) Combined hepatocellular-cholangiocarcinoma. A histologic and immunohistochemical study. Cancer 55: 124–135
15. Klatskin G (1965) Adenocarcinoma of the hepatic duct at its bifurcation within the porta hepatis. An unusual tumor with distinctive clinical and pathologic features. Am J Med 38: 241–256
16. Friedman AC, Sachs L, Birns MT (1987) Radiology of jaundice including choledocholithiasis and biliary neoplasms. In: Friedman AC (ed) Radiology of the liver, biliary tract, pancreas and spleen. pp 497–544
17. Takayasu K, Muramatsu Y, Moriyama N, Makuuchi M, Yamazaki S, Kishi K Yoshino M (1989) Hepatocellular and cholangiocellular carcinoma, double cancer of the liver: report of two cases resected synchronously and metachronously. Am J Gastroenterol 84(5): 544–547
18. Warren KW, Tan EGC (1975) Diseases of the gallblader and bile ducts. In: Schiff L (ed) Diseases of the Liver. Lippincott, Philadelphia, pp 1278–1335
19. Falk H, Thomas LB, Popper H, Ishak KG (1979) Hepatic angiosarcoma associated with androgenic anabolic steroids. Lancet 2: 1120–1123
20. Trotzke HA, Hutcheson JB (1965) Primary fibrosarcoma if the liver. South Med J 58: 236–238
21. Willis RA (1973) The spread of tumors in the human body. Butterworth, London
22. Netland PA, Zetter BR (1984) Organ-specific adhesion of metastatic tumor cells in vitro. Science 224: 1113–1115
23. Nicolson GL, Dulski KM (1986) Organ specificity of metastatic tumor colonization is related to organ-selective growth properties of malignant cells. Int J Cancer 38: 289–294
24. Van Rensburg SJ, Cook-Mozaffari P, Van Schalkwyk DJ, Van der Watt JJ, Vincent TJ, Purchase IF (1985) Hepatocellular carcinoma and dietary aflatoxin in Mozambique and Transkei. Br J Cancer 51: 713–726

3 Diagnosis and Staging of Malignant Liver Disease

Clinicians dealing with patients suspected of having malignant liver disease require answers to following questions: (a) Does the liver contain malignant liver lesions? Of which type? (b) Where are these lesions located? (c) Are these lesions resectable? (d) If the lesions are not resectable, can the patient be helped with interventional radiology?

The first question about the presence of malignant lesions can be answered by biochemical tests and by imaging techniques combined with a guided biopsy. Staging of detected lesions, which means localizing the lesions and assessing the resectability is a demanding but essential task for imaging techniques. Operable patients must be selected, and unnecessary exploratory laparotomies or laparoscopies can be avoided. Strengths and weaknesses of various detection or staging techniques are discussed below.

3.1 Clinical Aspects

3.1.1 Hepatocellular Carcinomas

Most patients have a history of liver disease such as acute or chronic hepatitis, cirrhosis, or increased intake of alcohol. In some countries and because of the presence of undiscovered non-A, non-B hepatitis viruses, blood transfusion is also noted in the history of patients with hepatocellular carcinoma. Presenting symptoms can be found in Fig. 3.1.

The clinical manifestation of hepatocellular carcinoma depends partially on the presence or absence of cirrhosis. In the absence of cirrhosis the general status remains good for a long time. Hepatocellular carcinoma can manifest with mass, with an acute abdomen (because of beginning rupture), with fever or be silent for a long period and found during a routine clinical follow-up for liver disease. Invasion or compression of biliary tracts causes obstructive jaundice and sometimes hemobilia presenting with colickly pain. Invasion of portal veins can lead to portal hypertension with subsequent variceal bleeding.

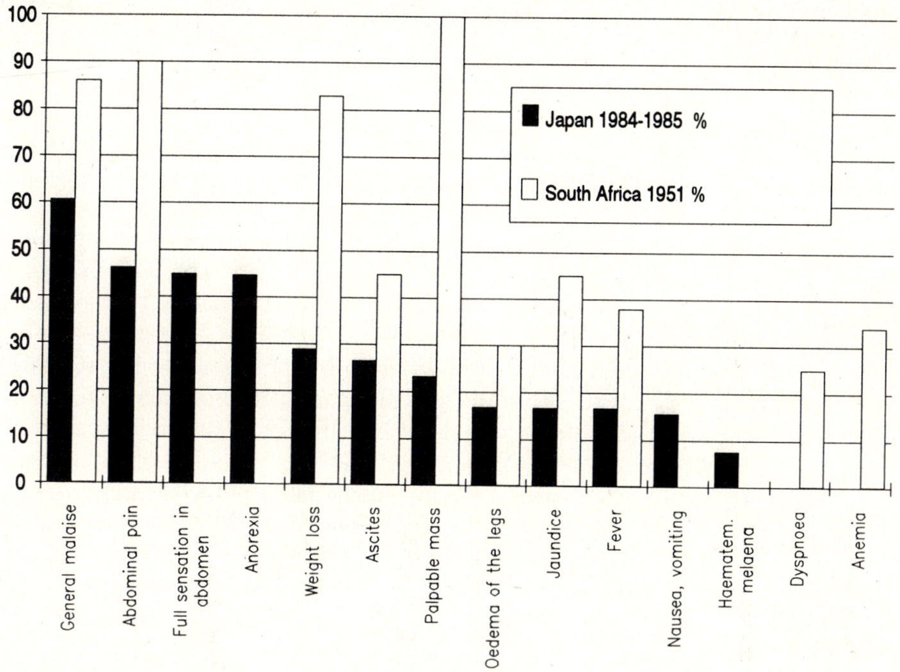

Fig. 3.1. Relative Frequency of early symptoms in patients with hepatocellular carcinoma in South Africa and Japan. (Complied from [1])

3.1.2 Metastases

Clinical manifestations of metastases depend on the extent of the disease. Metastases are almost always clinically silent at the beginning. As time passes and metastases grow, there is generally an alteration in the general status. Compression or invasion of bile ducts or compression by hilar lymphadenopathy causes obstructive jaundice. Metastases reaching the capsule may be painful: when tumors rub against the central part of the diaphragm, the pain is referred to the shoulders, whereas tumors rubbing against peripheral parts or the diaphragm cause pain at the site of the tumor. Hemorrhage within metastases can be felt as a painful episode related to distension of the liver capsule. Rupture of metastases with acute intraperitoneal bleeding is uncommon.

3.2 Biochemical Tests

Biochemical markers and hepatic function tests are helpful in the detection of malignant liver disease but lack sensitivity and specificity.

Screening for α-fetoprotein elevation uncovers about three fourths of hepatocellular carcinomas developing in patients with liver cirrhosis. In a series of 1738 patients with hepatocellular carcinoma only 18.9% had an α-fetoprotein level below 20 ng/ml whereas 76.9% of 117 patients with cholangiocarcinoma were below this level [2]. An α-fetoprotein value rising steeply over months appears more reliable than a fixed, preset threshold in detecting hepatocellular carcinoma [3]. A prospective study of 157 patients with confirmed cirrhosis showed that α-fetoprotein was less sensitive than ultrasound in detecting hepatocellular carcinomas but had predictive value. Patients with initial levels higher than 20 ng/ml developed a tumor within 2 years more frequently than patients with levels below 20 ng/ml [4].

In metastatic liver disease, elevation of alkaline phosphatase is frequently found, but the test is less sensitive and specific than ultrasound and CT [5]. In a prospective study of 48 patients with digestive carcinoma, elevation of alkaline phosphatase was shown to be less sensitive (50%) than elevation of γ-glutamyltransferase (86%) but more specific (96% against 88%) [6]. γ-Glutamyl-transferase is one of the most sensitive enzymes in detecting liver metastases, but its usefulness is greatest in the follow-up of therapy [7].

Carcinoembryonic antigen (CEA) is a glucoprotein that increases in the presence of intestinal tumors such as colon cancer and of liver metastases. Measuring α-fetoprotein and CEA is helpful for distinguishing hepatocellular carcinoma from metastases: high α-fetoprotein and low CEA levels favor a diagnosis of hepatocellular carcinoma. CEA is also important in the follow-up of metastatic liver disease.

Several other markers or isoenzymes such as variant alkaline phosphatase, α-L-fucosidase, transcobalamin, and des-γ-carboxy-prothrombin have been described. These tests have not yet reached widespread clinical significance.

Overall, modification of hepatic tests can give important clues for further investigations or imaging procedures; however, they lack sensitivity and specificity. The aphorism "negative values mean nothing" must be remembered.

3.3 Techniques in Imaging Malignant Liver Disease

3.3.1 Plain Film

Plain films of the abdomen are of limited value in the workup of malignant liver disease. Recognition of the right lateral liver margin and centralization of small bowel loops are signs indicating the presence of ascites. Calcifications in the liver are found in benign conditions such as hemangiomas, granulomatous infections, and parasitic infestations but also in association with malignant liver disease. Metastatic lesions in the liver calcify infrequently. In adults, metastases of colloid carcinoma of the rectum and colon are the lesions that most commonly calcify, but metastases of many other tumors may show the same behavior [8].

Calcification of primary carcinomas of the liver is unusual and occurs more commonly in children than in adults. Calcified primary malignant liver tumors are generally cholangiocarcinomas, cholangio-hepatocellular carcinomas, or fibrolamellar hepatocellular carcinomas in noncirrhotic young adults [9]. Discovery of irregular calcifications in the liver or detection of ascites must lead to further investigations with other imaging modalities such as ultrasound or CT.

3.3.2 Ultrasound

Conventional Ultrasound

The merits of ultrasound are manifold: ultrasound is cheap to perform and is readily available in most parts of the world. Its limitations are also well known: it is investigator-dependent and restricted by the presence of air in the acoustic window. The role of ultrasound consists in detection, localization, characterization, and assessment of spread of focal nodular lesions in the liver parenchyma. Its role consists further in detection of thrombosis of portal or hepatic veins and evaluation of operability.

Analysis of the echogenicity of detected lesions gives some clues on their nature. Anechoic lesions are considered to be cystic lesions. Presence of septa in anechoic lesions may suggest the diagnosis of hydatic disease. Hypoechoic lesions are generally malignant; bull's eye images seem characteristic for liver metastases. A variety of benign conditions, however, such as focal fatty infiltration, hemangioma, focal hepatitis, and liver abscesses can also present with hypoechoic liver lesions. Focal lesions due to nonneoplastic diseases such as cytomegalovirus lesions [10], tuberculosis [11], and porphyria [12] can be confused with liver metastases.

Hyperechoic lesions without dorsal enhancement correspond either to hypovascular metastases, commonly from the digestive tract, or to small hemangiomas. Hyperechoic lesions with dorsal enhancement and the presence of a segmental artery are found in metastases of endocrine or renal tumors. Hyperechoic lesions with dorsal enhancement and without the presence of a segmental artery are either metastases or benign lesions such as hemangiomas, adenomas, or focal nodular hyperplasia. Mixed echogenicity is found in a variety of conditions such as hepatocellular carcinoma, metastases, hemangioma, hepatic pseudotumors, and regenerative nodules [13].

Ultrasound contrast agents are under investigation. Injection of intraarterial CO_2 has shown results comparable to those of Lipiodol CT (see below) in the detection of small hepatocellular carcinoma [14].

Overall, ultrasound is a sensitive method for detection of liver lesions, with published sensitivity rates between 76% and 96%; the detection rate of hepatocellular carcinomas appears to be higher than that of liver metastases. Although the method is operator dependent, it is highly reproducible in trained hands.

Duplex Doppler–Color Doppler Ultrasound

The value of duplex Doppler ultrasound appears to be limited. In a series of 154 liver lesions [15] arterial Doppler signals were obtained within the body of the tumor, at its periphery, or in both locations from 86% of 63 hepatocellular carcinomas and at the periphery from 5 of 7 cholangiocarcinomas, 4 of 11 liver metastases, and 5 of 23 hemangiomas. No such signal was found in regenerative nodules or pseudotumors. The peak systolic shift was related to the degree of arterioportal shunting. Shunting is prominent in larger tumors but minor or non-existent in small hepatocellular carcinomas.

Color Doppler flow images can be useful in differential diagnosis of focal liver lesions, as hepatocellular carcinomas seem to have a characteristic aspect. In a series of 35 patients with malignant liver disease a "basket" pattern corresponding to a fine blood flow network surrounding a tumor nodule was noted in 75% of 20 hepatocellular carcinomas and was not seen in liver metastases. A detour pattern corresponding to a dilated portal vein meandering around the tumor mass was observed in liver metastases whereas color dots were found in central parts of hemangiomas [16].

Color Doppler ultrasound is a very useful modality for analysis of hepatic vasculature. With Doppler ultrasound the presence or absence of flow in the portal vein and its branches, the hepatic veins, or the inferior vena cava is easily assessed. It also permits flow quantification and detection of flow reversal. Complete portal thrombosis is detected by the absence of color signals whereas partial thrombosis is demonstrated by color signals molding the thrombus. Portal cavernoma is shown as multiple, small, colored vessels of different sizes in the hepatic pedicle.

In portal hypertension inversion of portal flow is detected immediately by the changing of the color of the signal. A decrease in the amplitude of the Doppler signal can be a sign of decrease in portal flow. Analysis of collateral circulation and detection of a repermeabilized umbilical vein is facilitated by Doppler ultrasound. Because of flow acceleration and turbulence, stenosis of the portal vein due to adenopathies can be recognized and distinguished from thrombosis.

Intraoperative Ultrasound

Intraoperative ultrasound is a very useful method as it combines the versatility and resolution of standard real-time ultrasound without being hindered by its drawbacks (no intestinal gas, no abdominal wall to penetrate). Intraoperative ultrasound is often decisive for the surgical strategy, sometimes modifying planned procedures. It contributes to a better assessment of tumor extent and helps to clarify the relationship of tumor to portal or hepatic veins [17]. Sometimes lesions undiscovered preoperatively are detected. Among all imaging techniques of the liver, intraoperative ultrasound is one of the most sensitive [18, 19], with a sensitivity of about 96% [20].

3.3.3 Computed Tomography

Since the early 1980s CT has undergone important technological improvements, with a remarkable increase in scanning speed and resolution. The excellent results obtained with conventional dynamic CT could be improved because of the development of new scanning techniques such as spiral CT, delayed scanning, CT portography, and Lipiodol scanning, all contributing to an increase in sensitivity and specificity.

In CT, detection of liver lesions depends on the difference in attenuation between lesion and liver parenchyma. Liver lesions may either be hypodense, isodense, or hyperdense in comparison to normal liver parenchyma. If sufficient difference in attenuation exists, lesions can be detected and located on plain CT by correctly adjusting window width and level. On unenhanced scans hepatocellular carcinomas may be recognized as hypodense lesions with an attenuation about 20–30 HU lower than adjacent liver parenchyma. Calcifications are rarely found in untreated tumors. Coarse, trabecular calcifications occupying the central part of the tumor are generally encountered in cholangiocarcinomas, fibrolamellar carcinomas, and mixed tumors. Metastases of mucinous adenocarcinomas may show punctate, dispersed calcifications (Fig. 3.2).

Dynamic CT Scanning

The difference in attenuation between the lesion and the normal liver parenchyma is, unfortunately, often too tenuous, and intravenous bolus injection of contrast media is necessary to increase the contrast. Contrast medium arrives in the liver in two peaks, an arterial peak and a portal venous peak. Blood supply to the liver is about 25% arterial and 75% portal in normal subjects, the proportion of portal blood supply being lower in patients with cirrhosis. Metastases and primary liver tumors receive most of their blood supply from the

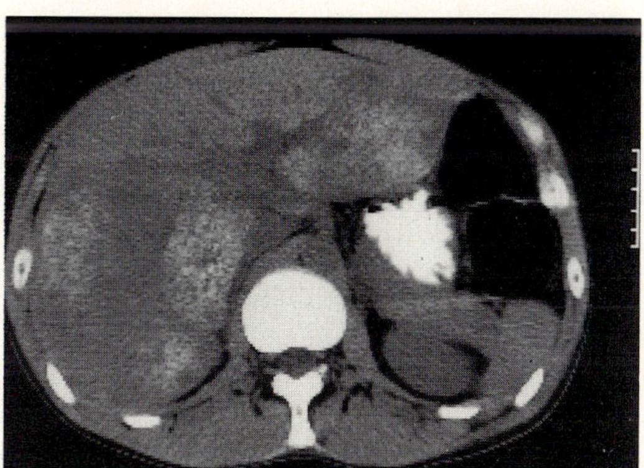

Fig. 3.2. Dispersed calcifications in metastases of mucinous adenocarcinoma of colon

hepatic arteries, portal veins having only a minor contribution. Due to the low proportion of arterial blood supply to normal liver parenchyma and the practically exclusive arterial blood supply to liver lesions the enhancement should be maximal in the first 20 s after injection of contrast material, before enhanced portal blood reaches the liver. Except for spiral CT scanners, most CT scanners are too slow and can only take one or two scans during this period. Most liver scanning occurs in a phase with maximum portal enhancement and in an equilibrium phase. To increase attenuation differences between normal liver parenchyma and liver lesions several injection protocols have been used, including drip infusions, infusions preceded by bolus injections or bolus injections alone. In our institution, we employ a biphasic protocol using a microprocessor-operated injector (Angiomat 6000, Liebel-Fleisheim, USA). A total of 150 ml contrast material (Ioxithalamate, Telebrix 300, Guerbet, France) is injected, first a bolus of 50 ml at a rate of 5 ml/s and then 100 cl at a slower rate of 2 ml/s, scanning beginning about 25 s after the beginning of injection.

Most metastases are hypodense and hypovascular. A high contrast between lesion and liver parenchyma is obtained by rapid scanning after injection of large doses of contrast material. Hepatocellular carcinomas generally show an irregular enhancement. Parts of the tumor may show the same enhancement pattern as normal liver and become obscured after contrast administration. Large doses of contrast material favor detection of venous invasion, which is encountered more often in hepatocellular carcinomas than in metastases.

Increasing contrast between tumor and normal liver parenchyma and thus visibility of the lesion is being investigated by several research groups. In CT, improvements can be expected soon in the field of new particulate contrast agents.

Conventional CT is a good imaging modality for detection of liver lesions. In a series of 929 patients with gynecological neoplasms, CT showed a sensitivity of 98% and specificity of 81% [21]. In another study in which CT was compared to other imaging modalities, CT demonstrated only 91 of 150 (61%) lesions in 54 patients undergoing resection surgery [22]. In a retrospective study on 100 patients with small hepatocellular carcinomas, dynamic CT showed a sensitivity of 84% [20]. A prospective study comparing the results of ultrasound and CT in 323 patients with liver tumors showed the high accuracy of ultrasound and CT, the sensitivity of ultrasound being 90.4% and that of CT 96.1% [23].

Delayed CT Scanning

Scanning 4–6 h after injection of large doses of contrast material (more than 60 g iodine) improves the detection rate of small liver lesions [24]. As 1%–2% of the iodinated contrast material is excreted through the liver in the biliary tract, normal liver parenchyma shows an enhancement of more than 20 HU in comparison to precontrast scans. In a series of 135 patients with liver metastases, delayed scanning permitted the detection of 13 lesions undiscovered with conventional contrast CT but missed 6 previously detected lesions. In any case, dynamic contrast CT and delayed scanning proved superior to precontrast scanning [25, 26]. Delayed scanning must be considered as a complementary method to dynamic CT and should be employed in patients with high risk of liver lesions having a normal dynamic CT study or when operability must be assessed. An important advantage of delayed scanning is that it is noninvasive.

CT Arteriography

CT arteriography is a method by which contrast is injected through a catheter into the hepatic artery, with dynamic scans being obtained in the arterial and early portal phases [27]. Small hepatocellular carcinomas, undiscovered tumor nodules, or hypervascular metastases may be detected with this method. Hypervascular vascular rims around lesions are also better displayed. CT arteriography is an expensive and invasive technique and should be reserved for patients evaluated for hepatic resection and in situations in which there is a discrepancy between different imaging modalities.

CT Portography

CT portography also combines angiography and CT. Contrast medium is injected into the superior mesenteric artery, and scans are obtained during the portal venous phase. As normal liver is supplied up to 75% by portal venous blood and neoplastic lesions up to 95% by arterial blood, normal liver parenchyma shows a strong enhancement whereas neoplastic lesions remain hypodense. Very tiny lesions are detected with this method. CT portography must be considered one of the most sensitive modalities in detecting tiny lever lesions.

CT portography is also most useful in assessing the extension of the tumor. Infiltration of tumor in portal structures is more easily detected, and the relationship of the tumor to structures of the porta hepatis is assessed with more precision than with standard CT (Fig. 3.3.).

A three-dimensional fast-reconstruction technique based on contiguous CT portography scans adds accuracy in determining the segmental location of hepatic metastases and improves preoperative assessment of resectability [28].

CT After Intraarterial Lipiodol Infusion

Lipiodol CT is also a combination of angiography and CT. About 5 ml Lipiodol (Guerbet, France), a contrast medium based on iodized poppy seed oil, is selectively injected into the hepatic artery through a catheter. The oily contrast medium is accumulated by the tumor, especially by hepatocellular carcinomas, whereas contrast medium in excess in the normal parenchyma is eliminated by macrophages and hepatic lymphatic drainage. Scans are obtained about 14 days after the injection. Lipiodol is often used as vector for chemotherapy and injected as an instable emulsion of contrast medium and doxorubicin or mytomycin C (see Chap. 8 about chemoembolization). Hepatocellular

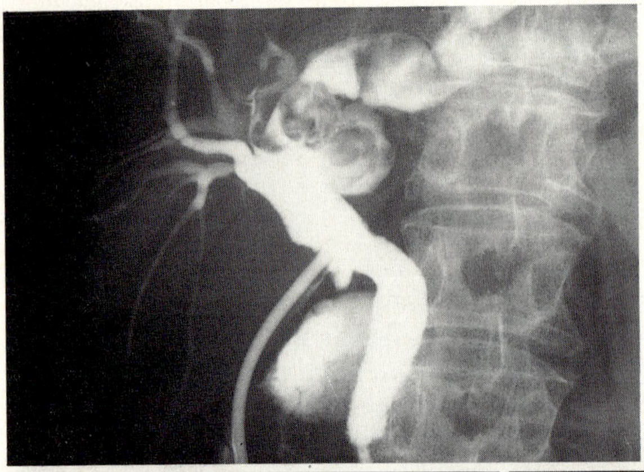

a

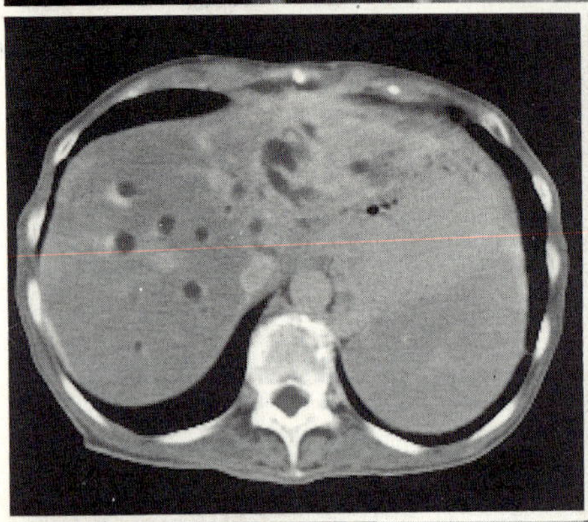

c

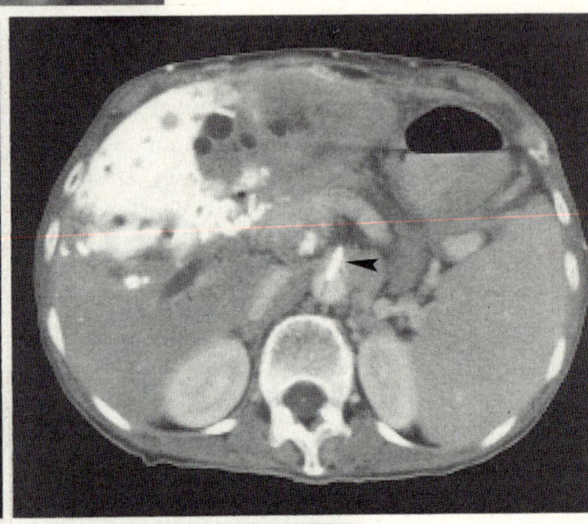

b

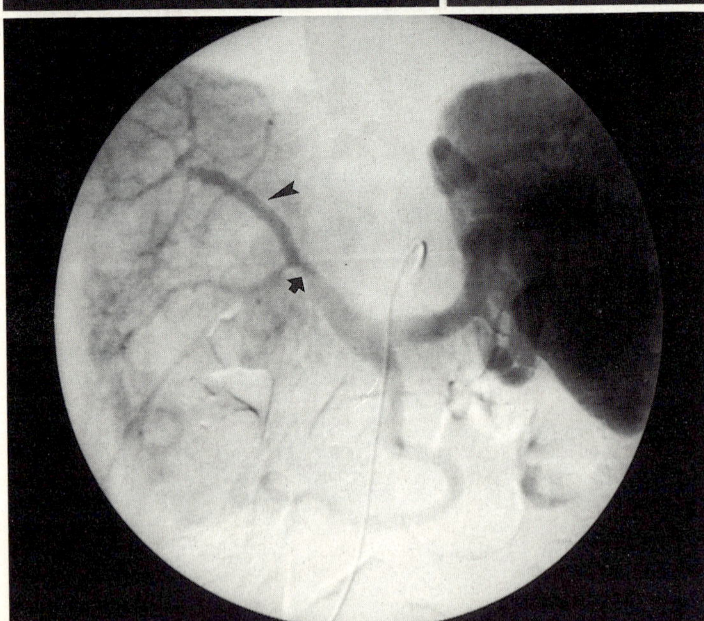

d

carcinomas and daughter nodules appear as high-density areas. This method can demonstrate very tiny lesion down to 5 mm in size and is generally employed to assess operability of known hepatic neoplasms as it is especially effective in detecting daughter nodules of hepatocellular carcinomas [29].

3.3.4 Magnetic Resonance

Until recently, MR suffered serious disadvantages in liver imaging: MR is an expensive technique that is not as widespread as ultrasound or CT, acquisition times are often too long, MR images lack sufficient spatial resolution, and they are deteriorated by different types of artifacts. The situation is changing. Newer sequences are appearing, allowing breath-hold imaging with acquisition times of some seconds. Acceptance is also increasing, and MR equipment is becoming more readily available. Although spatial resolution in the liver is far from that obtained in modern CT scans, the value of MR imaging resides in a richer image contrast between lesion and parenchyma. Using high-quality MR techniques it is now possible to display lesions below the 1-cm threshold [30, 31]. MR signal intensity ratios have been used to differentiate hemangiomas from metastases, high signal on late T2-weighted images typifying hemangiomas [32]. Using a T2 relaxation time greater than 88 ms and the presence of hyperintense morphology, Lombardo et al. [33] showed the possibility of distinguishing between hemangiomas and metastases.

New prospects are being opened by the development of contrast agents to increase the diagnostic yield of MR [34]. These contrast agents should provide information about tissue characterization and help to differentiate, for example, between vessels seen in cross-section and small tumors. The key issue for widespread use is drug tolerance. Pharmaceutical studies must still be completed.

Another field of investigation is the development of MR angiography for imaging of the abdominal vasculature, particularly the portal venous system. It is now possible [35] preoperatively to measure the flow and to assess the direction of flow in patients with cirrhosis to determine operability.

Still, at present time, the performance of MR is difficult to assess, as opinions about the comparative merits of MR and CT vary. Results concerning the

◄

Fig. 3.3 a–d. Patient with inoperable infiltrative cholangiocarcinoma. **a** Two years before CT examination, the patient had a cholecystectomy. The tumorous filling defects in T tube cholangiogram were interpreted by the surgeon in an outside hospital as blood clots. **b** Dynamic CT: enhancing tumorous tissue in left liver lobe and dilatation of bile ducts in both lobes. **c** CT portography. Catheter (*arrowhead*) lies in superior mesenteric artery. Strong contrast enhancement in superior mesenteric vein. Besides the strongly enhancing segment IV, there is little enhancement in other parts of the liver parenchyma, suggesting infiltration of portal veins and permeability of the vein irrigation segment IV. **d** Portal phase of selective arteriography of splenic artery. Note infiltration of portal main trunk (*arrow*) and absence of portal irrigation to left lobe. The thick intrahepatic vein (*arrowhead*) irrigates segment IV. Based on these findings the patient was considered inoperable and not treatable by chemoembolization

sensitivity and specificity of ultrasound, CT, and MR and especially the results of comparative studies should be interpreted with care. Variations in machine generation, different scanning techniques, comparison of brand-new technology with older machines, different expertise of the involved radiologist, and personal dedication of investigators to one technology introduce biases in studies comparing imaging modalities and influence their outcome. There are probably very few institutions dedicated to liver imaging that are able to compare the latest models of CT scanners and to perform, for example, spiral scanning, with the latest MR machines or high-end ultrasound devices. Clinical research lags behind technology.

Comparison of MR with recent CT techniques such as spiral scanning or spiral CT portography have still to be performed. With the advent of new sequences, new contrast agents, and use of high quality equipment, MR will undoubtedly become a very useful modality for liver imaging. It will probably be one of the methods to break through the "smaller than 1-cm barrier" in detection of neoplastic lesions.

3.3.5 Angiography

At present time angiography is seldom used as a pure diagnostic imaging modality, being supplanted by either ultrasound, CT or MR. Preoperatively, the use of angiography is essential in detailing vascular liver anatomy, assessing the blood supply of liver tumors, and detecting infiltration in major hepatic or portal vein. Angiography is still a useful technique in detecting small hypervascular metastases of endocrine tumors and in distinguishing hemangiomas from metastases. Due to the great variation in technique and angiographic skill of investigators, there is great variation in sensitivity of angiography in the detection of focal liver lesions. As a rule, hypervascular lesions are easier to pick up than hypovascular. Superselective catheterization provides more information than selective arteriography of the hepatic artery, and subtraction improves detection of lesions particularly in the left lobe (Figs 3.4, 3.5).

Angiography is often combined with other imaging modalities such as CT portography, CT arteriography, Lipiodol CT infusion, or interventional therapeutic procedures such as arterial chemotheraphy infusion or chemoembolization. Recent developments in catheter design, such as the catheter that we have developed (Hoogewoud superselective catheter, COOK, Denmark), and guide wire design permit superselective catheterization of small subsegmental arterial branches of the liver in patients in whom reaching the proper hepatic artery was not possible a few years ago. Digital subtraction angiography is a very useful technique in liver imaging and is increasingly replacing conventional arteriography. In comparison to conventional angiography, the lack of resolution of digital angiography is compensated by a greater sensitivity to contrast differences; liver parenchyma – especially the left liver lobe – and portal vessels are often shown more clearly. Digital fluoroscopy – an integral part of digital

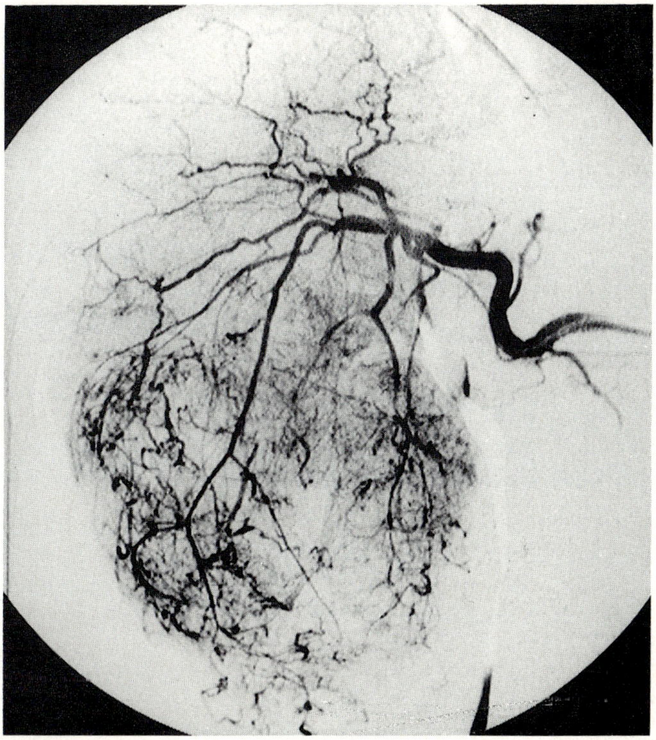

Fig. 3.4. Selective arteriography of right hepatic artery. Huge hypervascular hepatocellular carcinoma in segments V and VI

angiography – with facilities such as last image hold and reference image buffer are most helpful to the radiologists as it facilitates catheterization of small arteries, reduces radiation exposure of both patient and medical staff and speeds up the procedure. The lower film consumption of digital angiography helps reducing costs.

Splenoportography is most useful for investigating the portal venous system. Classically, the spleen is punctured with an 18-gauge cannula or catheter and 40 ml contrast media injected at a rate of 7 ml/s with a power injector. The examination can also be performed with a 22-gauge needle. Digital subtraction angiography may be helpful. Splenoportography provides fine images of the portal venous system and its collaterals. Measurements of portal venous pressure can be made (the normal pressure being 5–10 mmHg) and portal hypertension quantified. Provided that a good technique and fine needles are used, complications, especially hemorrhage, can be kept to a minimum. Embolization of the puncture tract with gelfoam particles further reduces the risk of complications.

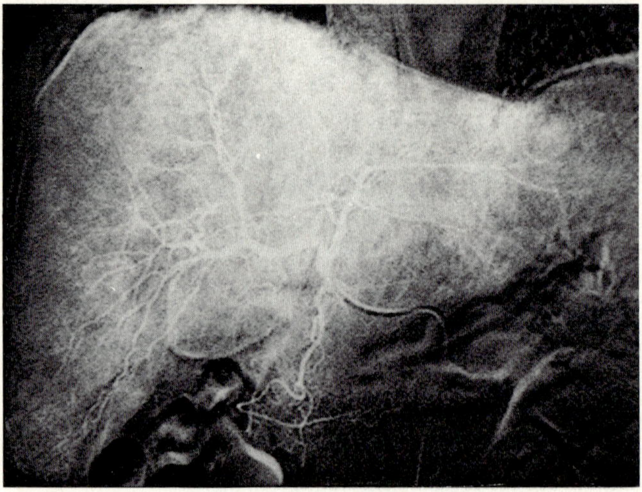

Fig. 3.5. Selective arteriography of common hepatic artery. Presence of countless tiny liver metastases of ovarian carcinoma. Note patchy nodularity of liver parenchyma

Transhepatic portography consists in percutaneous catheterization of the right portal vein through a right lateral intercostal puncture of the liver. A fine 23-gauge needle is used to reach the portal vein. A 0.014-inch guidewire is inserted, over which a catheter is placed in the portal vein. This technique is used for direct portography and selective catheterization of collaterals which might be occluded if sclerosing agents were used. Collaterals are precisely depicted and portal hypertension can also be precisely quantified by pressure measurements. This technique is also used for venous sampling when searching for a small endocrine tumor that has not been found with other imaging techniques such as CT, splanchnic arteriography, or scintigraphy.

Arteriography and splenoportography are generally not conclusive in the diagnosis of Budd-Chiari syndrome, which may be caused by thrombosis of hepatic veins (secondary to leukemia, *Aspergillus* invasion, senecio alkaloids, oral contraceptives, or trauma), by venous obstruction due to tumors such as hepatocellular carcinoma or metastases, by abscesses, or by webs, strictures, or membranes. Inferior vena cavography followed by selective catheterization of the hepatic veins provides detailed information of the cause of the syndrome. Webs, strictures, thrombi, or tumor invasion are precisely revealed and venous hepatic collaterals can be demonstrated.

3.3.6 Nuclear Medicine

In liver scintigraphy, metastases and hepatocellular carcinomas are manifested by either one or multiple areas of decreased activity or by an inhomogeneous distribution of the ^{99m}Tc-labeled sulfur colloid radionuclide within a normal or enlarged liver. The size of the smallest detectable lesion depends on the spatial resolution of the detecting system. With conventional techniques, lesions are best seen when located superficially, either anterior or posterior, and in the left lobe rather than in the right lobe. With single photon emission CT imaging, detection is less dependent on location. Some neoplasms, such as hepatomas, are gallium-67 avid and can be distinguished from pseudotumors that do not take up gallium-67. Both present as defects on the sulfur colloid images. Reported sensitivity in detection of malignant neoplastic liver lesions ranges between 60% and 100% and specificity between 67% and 100% [36]. Scintigraphic imaging of benign liver lesions or pseudotumors often helps to resolve the dilemma about the true nature of a detected lesion. Hemangiomas show increased activity on blood pool scans. Focal nodular hyperplasia and regenerating nodules are the only liver lesions containing sufficient numbers of Kupffer's cells to show an uptake of sulfur colloid equal to or greater than normal liver parenchyma. Exceptions to this rule exist. Liver cell adenomas are photopenic in sulfur colloid scintigraphy, as they are essentially devoid of Kupffer's cells but may show an activity in ^{99m}Tc-IDA scans. The concentration of this hepatobiliary tracer may be an expression of the ability of the adenoma to produce bile and its inability to excrete it due to a lack of functioning bile ducts. ^{99m}Tc-HIDA scans are used to assess permeability of the biliary tree.

Once a liver mass is found with scintigraphy, complementary examinations with ultrasound or CT are still necessary to distinguish whether a detected mass is liquid or solid, to examine the extent of the lesion, or to perform a guided biopsy. Clinicians are generally reluctant to stop investigations based on a normal scintigram if the clinical suspicion of liver metastases is high. Further, there are still considerable numbers of false-positive scintigram results due to defects from gallbladder, renal fossa, or porta hepatis. These disadvantages have led nuclear medicine to be replaced by other imaging modalities. Scintigraphy remains useful in imaging of suspected hemangiomas, focal nodular hyperplasia, and liver cell adenoma.

3.4 Imaging Malignant Focal Liver Lesions

3.4.1 Hepatocellular Carcinoma

Hepatocellular carcinomas vary in their morphological presentation as they can be solitary, multiple, or diffusely infiltrating. Diffusely infiltrating hepatocellular carcinomas can be difficult to detect.

Ultrasonography

The echogenicity of hepatocellular carcinoma nodules depends on their size and histological nature. Solid tumors without necrosis are generally hypoechoic.

Mixed echogenicity is found in tumors with partial necrosis. Fatty metamorphosis or sinusoidal dilatation makes tumors appear hyperechoic. Echogenicity may vary with size; small tumors may appear hypoechoic whereas larger tumors become hyperechoic. The fibrous capsule surrounding certain tumors may present as a hypoechoic halo. Depending on type of growth, tumors can present as clearly distinguishable nodule or as poorly defined parenchymal changes with a variety of echo patterns in the infiltrative type of tumors.

Computed Tomography

The most characteristic finding is an inhomogeneously enhancing mass on postcontrast dynamic scans. The tumor is often hypodense on precontrast scans; parts may become isodense to normal liver parenchyma, others show a strong enhancement on postcontrast scans. The inhomogeneity of enhancement is related to necrosis and variations in vascularization of the tumor. Fibrous capsules around hepatocellular carcinomas are found more often in Asian patients than in Caucasians.

Fast scanning during contrast injection may help to identify portal vein thrombosis or infiltration. Lobar hypodensity on precontrast scans can be the expression of fatty infiltration secondary to ischemia, portal vein density 20–30 HU lower than that of the aorta in the equilibrium phase, and dilatation of main portal vein or of lobar vein branches are signs of portal vein occlusion [37].

Biliary obstruction can be identified as dilatation of distal biliary ducts. In the absence of clear signs of malignancy such as vascular or biliary infiltration, differentiating solitary uncomplicated hepatocellular carcinomas from adenomas may be difficult, and biopsy is necessary. Hepatocellular carcinomas may be difficult to identify or even missed in patients with cirrhosis, especially when presenting as slightly hypodense lesions on precontrast scans showing only moderate or no enhancement on postcontrast scans. Suspect lesions should be biopsied.

3.4.2 Liver Metastases

Ultrasonography

Metastases show a variety of echogenicity patterns: anechoic, hypoechoic, hyperechoic, or mixed. Although tissue characterization is not possible, association between histology and echo patterns have been found. Metastases of colorectal cancers are often hyperechoic. Rapid growth of metastases, thus overgrowing vascularization, leads to necrosis and cystic degeneration. These changes can be seen, for example, in melanoma metastases which show changing appearances over time. Small lesions are generally hypoechoic. Later they develop echogenic centers with a hypoechoic halo. As the lesions enlarge, anechoic centers develop. Metastases of some necrotic tumors, such as leiomyosarcoma, may be anechoic. Lymphoma presents most frequently as hypoechoic masses with poor margin definition.

Echogenic foci with acoustic shadows are indicative for calcifications that are generally found in mucin-producing tumors such as colorectal cancer, bronchial cancer, and carcinomas of the ovary or breast.

Computed Tomography

The CT appearance of metastases shows extreme variations and depends on vascularization, size, histology, amount of necrosis, and patterns of diffusion of contrast medium in the interstitium. Metastases of different origin may have a similar presentation on CT scans and show as hyperattenuating or hypoattenuating lesions with a hyperattenuating rim. Hypoattenuating lesions with or without hyperattenuating rims are most common and are found in lung, breast, colon, and pancreas cancer. Hyperattenuating rims reflect vascularization of viable tumor periphery contrasting with the necrotic center. Because of hepatic arterial supply these rims are best seen after hepatic artery administration of contrast or in early scans when a large dose of contrast is injected intravenously at a high rate.

Hyperattenuating lesions are uncommon and found in metastases of neuroendocrine tumors, and renal and thyroid cancer.

Tumors may be hardly detectable when they are nearly isodense to normal liver on precontrast scans and show only little enhancement on postcontrast scans. They may, however, be seen on delayed CT scans or with CT portography.

Detection of lesions can be difficult in livers presenting with diffuse or geographic fatty infiltration, such as after chemotherapy or intravenous alimentation. Normal liver parenchyma presents as a "negative" with parenchyma having a lower attenuation number than vessels on precontrast scans. In these cases metastases may become hyperattenuating on postcontrast scans. Perifocal rims are also better seen because of better contrast to the fatty liver and the necrotic center.

3.4.3 Cholangiocarcinoma

Infiltrating cholangiocarcinoma is difficult to detect by ultrasonography or CT. Dilatation of bile ducts can easily be recognized but the obstructing mass is rarely recognized or difficult to demarcate as it blends with hilar structures (Fig. 3.3a). Percutaneous transhepatic cholangiography is helpful in recognizing infiltration of the bile ducts and localizing the site and nature of the obstruction. It is also helpful in guiding intrabiliary biopsies, for example, with an atherotomy catheter.

Some cholangiocarcinomas are peripheral intrahepatic tumors that may be multifocal and mimic hepatocellular carcinoma or metastases.

3.4.4 Lymphoma

In most hepatic manifestations of lymphoma there is a diffuse infiltration of periportal tracts. Besides hepatomegaly, no abnormal feature can be found with imaging techniques. Core biopsy yields the diagnosis. In patients with acquired immunodeficiency syndrome lymphoma may present with a multifocal nodular manifestation. Hypoattenuating masses, which may have enhancing rims, can be found in liver, spleen, and kidney. Metastases of Kaposi's sarcoma or other primary cancers and multiple hepatic abscesses belong to the differential diagnosis.

3.4.5 Fatty Infiltration

Fatty infiltration of the liver, which can be focal, geographic, or diffuse, may mimic metastases, a primary hepatic tumor, or infarction. It is commonly found in oncology patients after chemotherapy. Intravenous alimentation, alcoholism, obesity, diabetes, and hypertriglyceridemia are other frequent causes. Focal fatty infiltration can also be secondary to portal infiltration or hepatic infarction. It is a reversible condition, depending on diet or drug therapy.

In ultrasonography, the presentation of diffuse fatty liver depends on the extent of the infiltration. Mild infiltration presents as a slight increase of the echogenicity of the liver parenchyma. The visualization of intrahepatic vessels and diaphragm is impaired in moderate infiltration. In marked infiltration the vessels and the diaphragm may be indistinguishable due to attenuation and scattering of sound. Focal fatty liver may present as poorly defined, hyperechoic lesions mimicking metastases or hepatocellular carcinoma.

In CT the attenuation of normal liver parenchyma is normally 5–10 HU greater than that of spleen on precontrast scans. Fatty infiltration is present when the attenuation of liver is lower than that of a normal spleen. Attenuation values of fatty liver may reach water equivalent or negative values. In CT the appearance of focal fatty liver also causes a diagnostic dilemma because it can mimic liver cancer. Recognizing normal vessels following an undistorted course through the focal lesions strongly favors the diagnosis of focal fatty liver. Doubtful lesions must be biopsied.

MR using fat suppression or fat and water suppression techniques is helpful in distinguishing focal fatty infiltration from tumor.

3.5 Percutaneous Liver Biopsy

Using imaging techniques, the diagnosis of the nature of lesions can be made and is based on appearance, clinical context, experience, statistics, and probability. Frequently, however, the exact nature of a lesion must be determined, and assumptions are not good enough ("CT does not replace the microscope!"). So called "specific" echogenicity, contrast enhancement patterns or T2 relaxation times are characteristics that can be shared by a variety of lesions, either benign or malignant.

3.5.1 Biopsy of Malignant Liver Lesions

CT- or ultrasound-guided biopsies are very valuable methods (Fig. 3.6.). In a series about 441 controlled cases, ultrasound-guided fine needle aspiration biopsy using a 22-G Chiba needle was performed. Specificity was 100%, sensitivity 93.2%, and overall accuracy 95%. CT and ultrasound are equally effective in providing diagnostic material [38]. There is still controversy as to whether large needles (14 or 18-G) should be preferred to fine needles (21 or 22-G). In a study comparing 22-G needles with 18-G needles, higher sensitivity in the diagnosis of malignant disease (18-G, 91.2%, 22-G, 71.4%) and in distinguishing between primary and secondary malignant tumor (18-G, 86.5%; 22-G, 42.9%) favored the use of large needles [39], whereas in another study comparing coarse-needle biopsy (14-G) versus fine-needle biopsy (22-G) equally satisfying results were found with the two techniques [40]. False-positive diagnosis of malignancy is an extreme rarity, and published specificity of guided liver biopsy is invariably 100%. In our own series of liver biopsies we also have a specificity of 100%. Examples of biopsies are shown in Figs 3.7–3.11.

Results of guided fine-needle aspiration biopsy depend on the technical skills of the radiologist, which comprise exact localization of the needle in the tumor and correct aspiration technique in order to obtain sufficient material of good quality for analysis. A close collaboration with the laboratory performing the morphological examination is mandatory, especially with regard to accurate processing of the aspirated material.

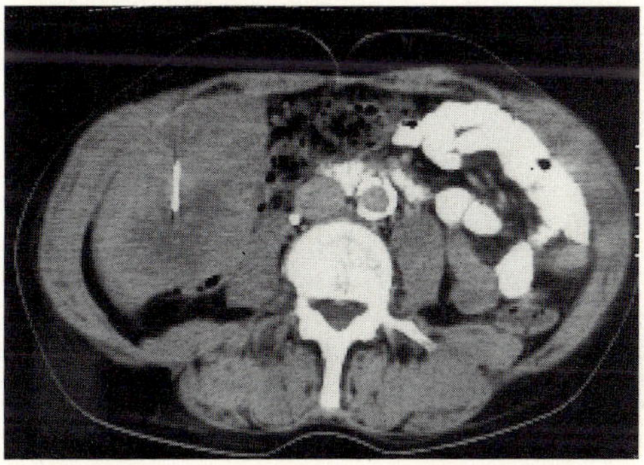

Fig. 3.6. CT-guided fine-needle aspiration biopsy of hepatocellular carcinoma. Needle tip is located at border in viable part of tumor, thus avoiding the often encountered tumor necrosis of central parts

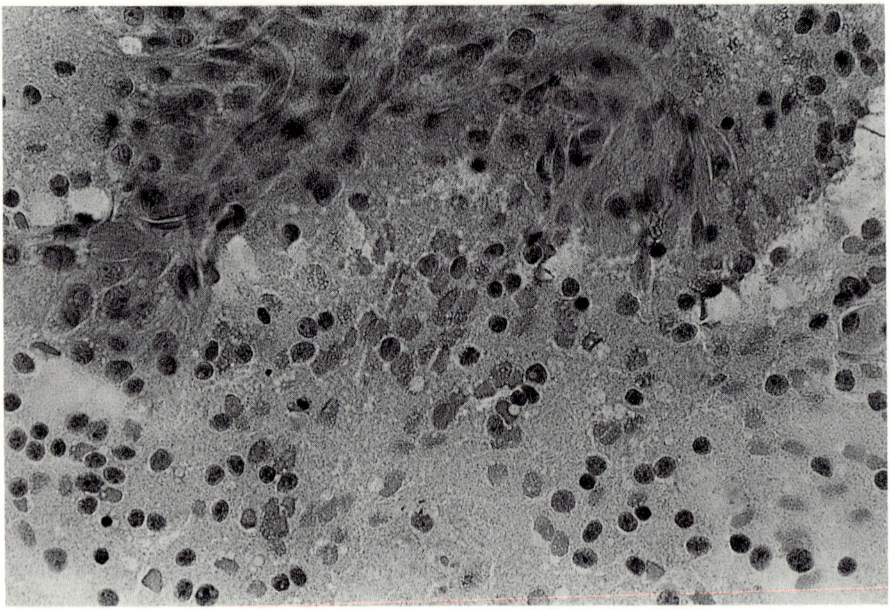

Fig. 3.7. Patient: m. 71y. Fine needle aspiration biopsy of a tumor in the right hepatic lobe. Clusters and isolated cells ("naked nuclei") of a hepatocellular carcinoma; Papanicolaou, ×350

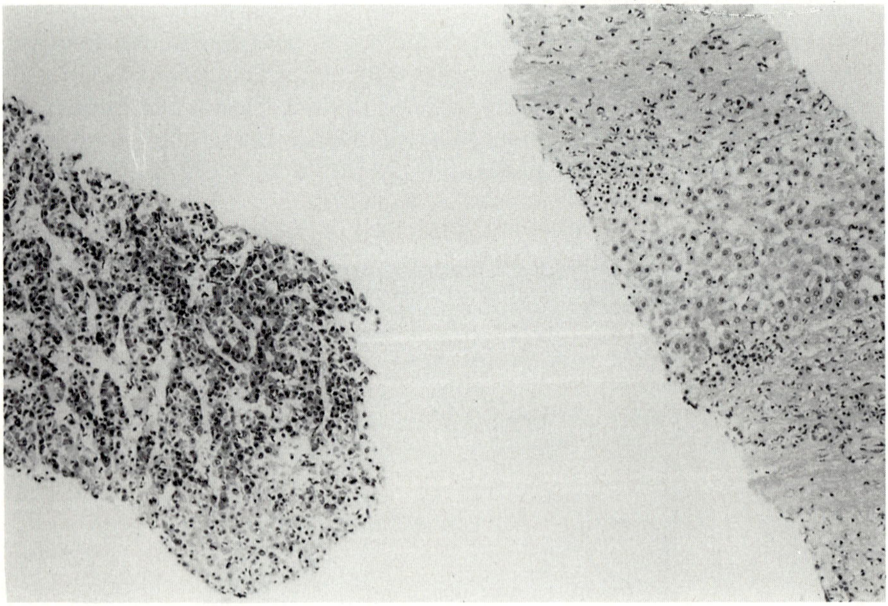

Fig. 3.8. Same patient as Fig. 3.7. Two fragments of hepatic biopsy containing hepatic parenchyma suggestive of micronodular cirrhosis (left) and hepatocellular carcinoma (right; trabecular type, grade 2 [Edmonson and Steiner]). H&E, ×88

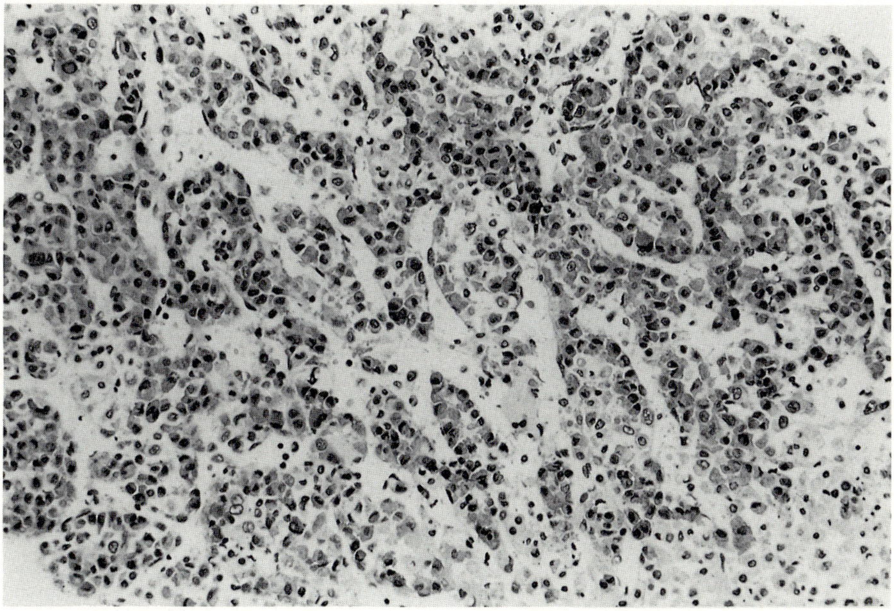

Fig. 3.9. Same patient as Fig. 3.7 and Fig. 3.8. Higher magnification of hepatocellular carcinoma (trabecular type, grade 2 [Edmonson and Steiner]). H&E, ×175

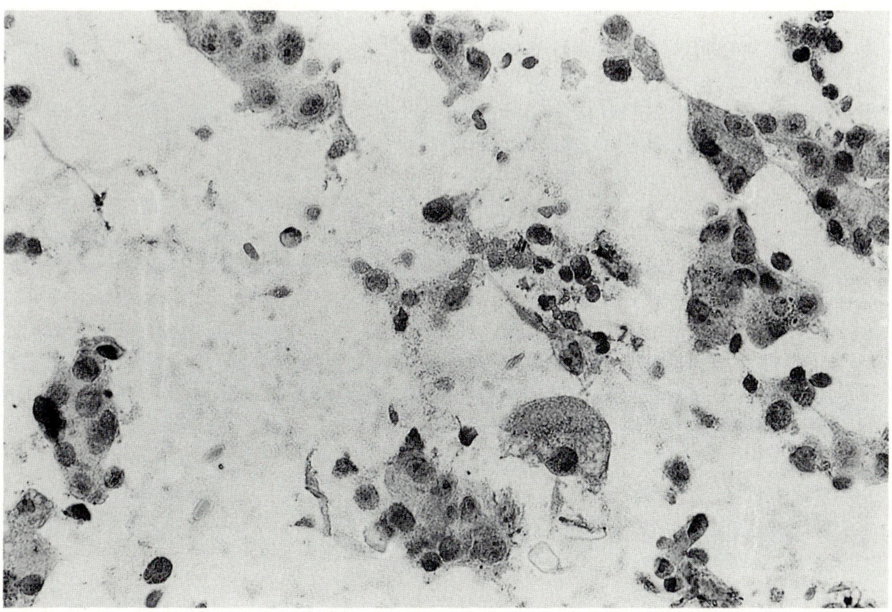

Fig. 3.10. Patient: f. 72y. Fine needle aspiration biopsy with some degenerated hepatocytes and clusters of metastatic carcinoma. Papanicolaou, ×350

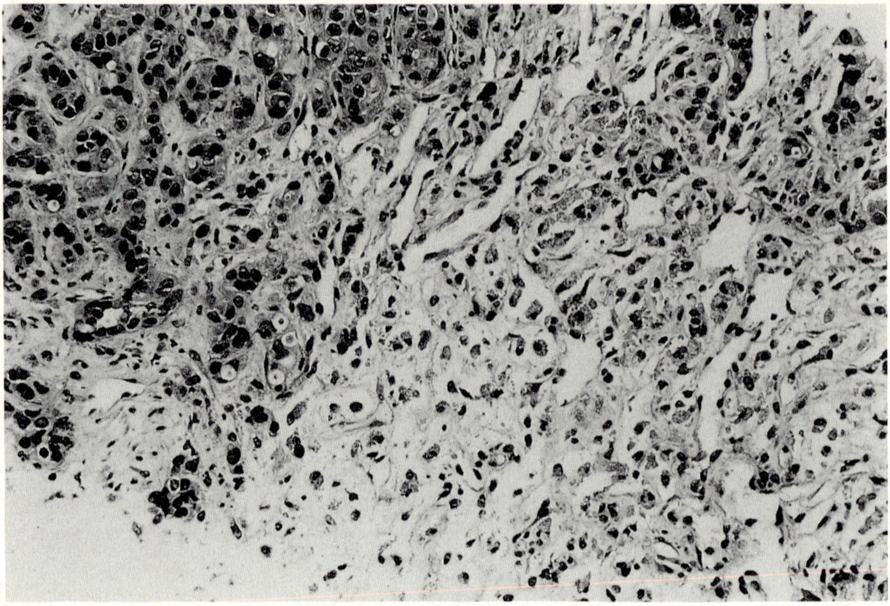

Fig. 3.11. Same patient as Fig. 3.10. Hepatic biopsy with atrophic hepatic parenchyma and metastasis of a poorly differentiated, trabecular carcinoma; a mammary carcinoma of the same morphologic type was detected simultaneously. H&E, ×175

3.5.2 Biopsy of Liver Hemangiomas

Not too long ago, biopsying a hemangioma was considered taboo because of the risk of bleeding. Although hemangiomas have typical presentations in various imaging modalities, confusion with malignant lesions still frequently occurs as atypical hemangiomas can perfectly mimic malignant lesions. Numerous lesions biopsied in the belief that they were metastases were shown in fact to be hemangiomas, and the complication rate was not as high as expected. Patients and clinicians need certitude and cannot be satisfied, for example, with an 85% chance of a hemangioma. Thus biopsy of hemangiomas may be warranted as the presence of malignant lesions may be excluded and the diagnosis of hemangiomas made positively [41]. Care must be taken to choose a needle path through healthy liver before entering the lesion to avoid bleeding (Fig. 3.12).

3.5.3 Complications of Biopsy

Complications of guided needle biopsy are very rare. In a series about 350 patients on whom percutaneous CT-guided biopsies using needles of various diameters were carried out, complications that did not require treatment

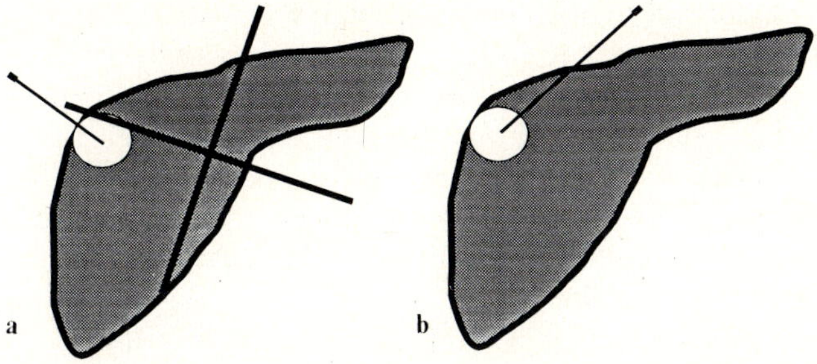

Fig. 3.12. a Wrong way to biopsy superficial hypervascular lesions or hemangiomas. Danger of hemorrhage! **b** Correct way. Needle should pass first through healthy liver parenchyma before entering the lesion

occurred in five patients (1.4%) [42]. Bleeding, needle tract seeding, and infection are the most frequently cited complications. Bleeding occurs most frequently when a hypervascular lesion such as a hemangioma, hemangiosarcoma [43], or hepatoma is biopsied. The risk of bleeding can be lowered if the needle enters first a layer of 2-3 cm of unaltered liver tissue before entering the lesion, as normal liver tissue may function as a tamponade. When biopsy is performed through a sleeve, the needle tract may be embolized with Gelfoam particles, such as in the spleen after splenoportography [44]. In a personal case an important hemorrhage due to needle laceration of the liver occurred after biopsy of a hepatoma in an alcoholic patient who exhaled instead of holding his breath. Needle track recurrence is infrequent and is generally reported anecdotally [45]. Mortality rate with fine-needle biopsy is about 0.036%–0.1% and is most often due to hemorrhage [46–48] or infection [49]. A fatal carcinoid crisis after percutaneous fine-needle biopsy of liver metastases has also been described [50]. Overall, percutaneous liver biopsy must be considered as a safe procedure with low rate of complications and mortality with proper technique and careful patient selection.

3.6 Principles of Staging of Liver Lesions

Indications and contraindications of various therapeutic modalities, discussed in other chapters, rely heavily on the accuracy of staging, which is based on the presence, number, localization, and nature of liver lesions and the determination of resectability. Liver lesions must be localized precisely in the different liver segments; safe distance to main vascular trunks must be assessed; and invasion of portal veins, hepatic veins, or biliary radicles and neoplastic arteriovenous fistulas must be recorded. Ultrasound, CT, and MR are very useful in segmental localization of liver lesions. Locating lesions situated at the borders of two segments may be difficult, especially with CT. Due to the transverse separation plane, it can be difficult to distinguish between segments II and III, V and VIII, and VI and VII. It is easier to follow the vascular landmarks in all the planes with ultrasound; therefore it can be considered as the method of choice for localization. Invasion of portal veins is well detected by ultrasound, angiography, CT, and MR. Invasion of hepatic veins is best seen with ultrasound, angiography, and MR. Arteriovenous fistulas are best detected with angiography or bolus-enhanced CT. Obstruction of the biliary tree can be caused by compression of tumor masses or hilar adenopathies or by direct tumor invasion in the biliary ducts. Ultrasound, CT, or MR can generally described the cause of the extrinsic compression; direct invasion is, however, more difficult to assess and percutaneous transhepatic cholangiography must be performed in selected cases.

3.7 Which Method to Choose?

Detection of liver lesions should be carried out with ultrasound or CT. Depending on the organization of the imaging department, delayed scanning with CT may be performed systematically or in selected cases. MR may help to determine the nature of a lesion. Screening cirrhotic patients for the presence of hepatoma should be performed preferably with a combination of ultrasound and measurement of α-fetoprotein. Duplex or color Doppler ultrasound are useful in analyzing the vascularity and vascular complications of malignant liver lesions.

Unclear lesions should be biopsied as no imaging modality gives certitude about the nature of a lesion. The risk of the procedure is outweighed by far by the advantage of having a morphological diagnosis.

Basic staging of liver lesions should be performed with ultrasound and CT. If this staging shows the lesion to be potentially operable, further investigations must be performed. CT portography or MR might show further undetected lesions, and angiography demonstrates the anatomy and possibly the presence of previously undetected vascular involvement by the tumor. In the presence of a potentially operable hepatoma, Lipiodol CT may help to detect daughter nodules that may render the tumor inoperable, depending on their location. The disadvantage of the method is the delay between injection of Lipiodol and scanning.

References

1. Okuda K, Okuda H (1991) Primary liver cell carcinoma. In: McIntyre N, Benhamou JP, Bircher J, Rizetto M, Rodes J (eds) Oxford textbook of clinical hepatology. Oxford University Press, Oxford.
2. The Liver Cancer Study Group of Japan (1987) Primary liver cancer in Japan. Sixth report. Cancer 60: 1400–1417

3. Arrigoni A, Andriulli A, Gindro T, Piantino P, Capussotti L, Rizzetto M (1988) Pattern analysis of serum alpha-fetoprotein in the early diagnosis of hepatocellular carcinoma in liver cirrhosis. Int J Biol Markers 3: 172–176
4. Cottone M, Turri M, Caltagirone M, Maringhini A, Sciarrino E, Virdone R, Fusco G, Orlando A, Marino L, Pagliaro L (1988) Early detection of hepatocellular carcinoma associated with cirrhosis by ultrasound and alpha-fetoprotein: a prospective study. Hepatogastroenterology 35: 101–103
5. Schillinger H, Traeder R, Klosa W, Pohl J (1988) Nachweis von Lebermetastasen gynäkologischer Malignome durch Sonographie, Szintigraphie, Computertomographie und Leberenzyme. Onkologie 11: 216–220
6. Osanaga E, Larre-Borges A, Sanguinetti J, Mancusso G, Lopez A, Larreborges U (1985) Comparative study between alkaline phosphatase and gamma-glutamyltranspeptidase in the diagnosis of hepatic metastases. J Chir (Paris) 122: 17–20
7. Külling D, Sauter C (1990) Die Bedeutung der γ-Glutamyltransferase zur Erfolgsbeurteilung einer Chemotherapie von Lebermetastasen. Schweiz Med Wochenschr 120: 1435–1438
8. Darlak JJ, Moskowitz M, Kattan KR (1980) Calcifications in the liver. Radiol Clin North Am 18: 214
9. Friedman AC, Fishman EK, Radecki PD, Scatarige JC, Sherman JL, Farmlett EJ, Markle BM, Dachman AH, Pakter RL (1987) Focal diseases. In: Friedman AC (ed) Radiology of the liver, biliary tract, pancreas and spleen, Baltimore p 222
10. Vieco PT, Rochon L, Lisbona A (1990) Multifocal cytomegalovirus-associated hepatic lesions simulating metastases in AIDS. Radiology 176: 123–124
11. Belloir A, Guiry P, Guiry M, Maubon A, Rouanet JP, Bruel JM, Lamarque JL (1988) Tuberculose hépatique pseudo-tumorale. Aspects échographiques et scanographiques à propos d'un cas. J Radiol 69: 21–23
12. Kersjes W, Harder T, Steudel A, Hartlapp JH (1988) Multiple Leberrundherde bei latenter Porphyria cutanea tarda. ROFO 148: 165–168
13. Taboury J (1989) Echographie abdominale. Masson, Paris, pp 35–80
14. Kudo M, Tomita S, Tochio H, Mimura J, Okabe Y, Kashida H, Hirasa M, Ibuki Y, Todo A (1992) Small hepatocellular carcinoma: diagnosis with US angiography with intraarterial CO_2 microbubbles. Radiology 182: 155–160
15. Ohnishi K, Nomura F (1989) Ultrasonic Doppler studies of hepatocellular carcinoma and comparison with other hepatic focal lesions. Gastroenterology 97: 1489–1497
16. Tanaka S, Kitamura T, Fujita M, Nakanishi K, Okuda S (1990) Color Doppler flow imaging of liver tumors. AJR Am J Roentgenol 154: 509–514
17. Salminen PM, Hockerstedt K, Edgren J, Scheinin TM, Tierala E (1990) Intraoperative ultrasound as an aid to surgical strategy in liver tumor. Acta Chir Scand 156: 329–332
18. Parker GA, Lawrence W Jr, Horsley JS III, Neifeld JP, Cook D, Walsh J, Brewer W, Koretz MJ (1989) Intraoperative ultrasound of the liver affects operative decision making. Ann Surg 209: 569–576
19. Holscher AH, Stadler J (1989) Intraoperative Sonographie zum Nachweis occulter Lebermetastasen beim colorectalen Carcinom. Langenbecks Arch Chir 374: 363–369
20. Takayasu K, Moriyama N, Muramatsu Y, Makuuchi M, Hasegawa H, Okazaki N, Hirohashi S (1990) The diagnosis of small hepatocellular carcinomas: efficacy of various imaging procedures in 100 patients. AJR Am J Roentgenol 155: 49–54
21. Schillinger H, Traeder R, Klosa W, Pohl J (1988) Nachweis von Lebermetastasen gynäkologischer Malignome durch Sonographie, Szintigraphie, Computertomographie und Leberenzyme. Onkologie 11: 216–220
22. Clarke MP, Kane RA, Steele G Jr, Hamilton ES, Ravikumar TS, Onik G, Clouse ME (1989) Prospective comparison of preoperative imaging and intraoperative ultrasonography in the detection of liver tumors. Surgery 106: 849–855
23. Hruby W, Traxler M, Wassipaul M, Stellamor K (1988) Vergleich zwischen Ultraschall- und CT-Diagnostik solider Lebertumoren. ROFO 148: 378–383

24. Bernadino ME, Erwin BC, Steinberg HV, Baumgartner BR, Torres WE, Gedgaudas-McClees RK (1986) Delayed hepatic CT-scanning: increased confidence and improved detection of hepatic metastases. Radiology 159: 71–74
25. Bruneton JN, Rogopoulos A, Merran D, François E, Balu-Maestro C, Geoffray A, Cambon P, Bittman O (1990) Scanographie hépatique. Utilité des coupes tardives (6 heures) chez des patients ayant une fonction biliaire normale. J Radiol 71: 271–277
26. Freeny PC, Marks WM (1983) CT arteriography of the liver. Radiology 148: 193–197
27. Prando A, Wallace S, Bernardino ME, Lindell NM (1979) Computed tomographic arteriography of the liver. Radiology 130: 697–701
28. Soyer P, Roche A, Gad M, Shapeero L, Breittmayer F et al. (1991) Preoperative segmental localization of hepatic metastases: utility of three-dimensional CT during arterial portography. Radiology 180: 653–658
29. Ohishi H, Uchida H, Ohue S, Yoshimura H, Yoshioka T, Matsuo N, Yoshida H, Fukai Y (1988) Computed tomography detection of small daughter nodules in hepatocellular carcinoma after iodized oil infusion into the hepatic artery. J Comput Tomogr 12: 129–134
30. Vlachos L, Trakadas S, Gouliamos A, Lazarou S, Mourikis D, Ioannou R, Kalovidouris A, Papavasiliou C (1990) Comparative study between ultrasound, computed tomography, intraarterial digital subtraction angiography, and magnetic resonance imaging in the differentiation of tumors of the liver. Gastrointest Radiol 15: 102–106
31. Ward BA, Miller DL, Frank JA, Dwyer AJ, Simmons JT, Chang R, Shawker TH, Choyke P, Chang AE (1989) Prospective evaluation of hepatic imaging studies in the detection of colorectal metastases: correlation with surgical findings. Surgery 105: 180–187
32. Stark DD, Felder RC, Wittenberg J et al. (1985) Magnetic resonance imaging of cavernous hemangiomas of the liver. AJR Am J Roentgenol 145: 213–222
33. Lombardo DM, Baker ME, Spritzer CE, Blinder R, Meyers W, Herfkens RJ (1990) Hepatic hemangiomas vs metastases: MR differentiation at 1.5 T. AJR Am J Roentgenol 155: 55–59
34. Hamm B, Vogl TJ, Branding G, Schnell B, Taupitz M, Wolf KJ, Lissner J (1992) Focal liver lesions: MR imaging with MN-DPDP – initial clinical results in 40 patients. Radiology 182: 167–174
35. Hoogewoud HM, Edelman RR, Mattle H, Terrier F, Vock P (1990) Angiographie par résonance magnétique. Schweiz Med Wochenschr 1598–1607
36. Oppenheim BE, Wellman HN, Hoffer PB (1988) Liver imaging. In: Gottschalk A, Hoffer PB, Potchen EJ (eds) Diagnostic nuclear medicine, vol 2. Williams and Wilkins, Baltimore, pp 538–595
37. Mathieu D, Grenier P, Larde D, Vasile N (1984) Portal vein involvement in hepatocellular carcinoma: dynamic CT features. Radiology 152: 127–132
38. Butler JA, Smith C (1989) Fine-needle aspiration biopsy in the diagnosis of recurrent and metastatic intraabdominal malignancies. Am J Surg 158: 589–592
39. Seitz JF, Giovannini M, Monges G, Rosello R, Hassoun J, Mazel C, Gauthier A (1990) Etude comparative de la cytologie à l'aiguille fine et de la biopsie à l'aiguille de fort calibre sous contrôle échographique dans le diagnostic des tumeurs abdominales. Gastroenterol Clin Biol 14: 529–533.
40. Bedenne L, Mottot C, Courtois B, Meny B, Cauvin JM, Hillon P, Michiels R, Klepping C (1990) L'aiguille Tru-Cut est-elle plus efficace que l'aiguille fine dans le diagnostic des lésions hépatiques? Etude comparative de 45 ponctions guidées par l'échographie. Gastroenterol Clin Biol 14: 62–66
41. Taavitsainen M, Airaksinen T, Kreula J, Paivansalo M (1990) Fine-needle aspiration biopsy of liver hemangioma. Acta Radiol 31: 69–71
42. Feuerbach S, Gmeinwieser J, Gerhardt P, Gossner W, Rotter M, Gossmann A (1989) CT-gesteuerte Biopsie–Methoden, Resultate und Komplikationen. ROFO 151: 4–9
43. Hertzanu Y, Peiser J, Zirkin H (1990) Massive bleeding after fine needle aspiration of liver angiosarcoma. Gastrointest Radiol 15: 43–46
44. Probst P, Rysavy JA, Amplatz K, (1978) Improved safety of splenoportography by plugging of the needle tract. AJR Am J Roentgenol 131: 445–449

45. Scheele J, Altendorf-Hofmann A (1990) Tumor implantation from needle biopsy of hepatic metastases. Hepatogastroenterology 37: 335–337
46. Terriff BA, Gibney RG, Scudamore CH (1990) Fatality from fine-needle aspiration biopsy of a hepatic hemangioma (Letter). AJR Am J Roentgenol 154: 203–204
47. Weiss H, Weiss A, Scholl A (1988) Tödliche Komplikation einer Feinnadelbiopsie der Leber. Dtsch Med Wochenschr 113: 139–142
48. Gebel M, Horstkotte H, Koster C, Brunkhorst R, Brandt M, Atay Z (1986) Ultraschallgezielte Feinnadelpunktion abdomineller Organe: Indikationen, Ergebnisse, Risiken. Ultraschall Med 7: 198–202
49. Howard JM, Campbell EW (1989) Fatal clostridial pancreatitis following ERCP and percutaneous needle biopsy. Int J Pancreatol 5: 305–310
50. Bissonnette RT, Gibney RG, Berry BR, Buckley AR (1990) Fatal carcinoid crisis after percutaneous fine-needle biopsy of hepatic metastasis: case report and literature review. Radiology 174: 751–752

4 Surgical Treatment of Malignant Liver Lesions

4.1 Liver Resection

Healthy liver parenchyma has the unique capacity for regeneration. Resection of up to about 80% of noncirrhotic liver parenchyma is compatible with life. Remaining liver cells become larger, undergo increased mitosis, and rapidly replace missing parenchyma. Resection surgery should be complete with curative intention, leaving in place only healthy liver tissue. Resection surgery is still considered the single best treatment of neoplastic liver lesions.

4.1.1 Criteria for Resection

Role of Imaging

Imaging techniques play a crucial role preoperatively in the diagnosis, selection, and staging of tumors to be excised. Knowledge of the location of lesions in relation to major anatomical landmarks helps the surgeon to take adequate intraoperative measures to avoid surgical disasters. Because of extension, some patients are spared unnecessary surgery. Knowledge of the location of tumors can also increase the number of candidates for surgery as tumors located, for instance, in both lobes but caudal to the transverse plane can also be resected. Ideally, radiologists should be able to localize the tumors on a scheme of the liver to show the surgeon the relationship of the lesion to the various anatomical landmarks.

Vessels

Preoperatively, the relation of vital structures such as the main portal trunk, the vena cava, and the confluence between the hepatic veins and vena cava to the tumor must be assessed precisely. As a principle, invasion of one of these structures renders lesions nonresectable. Invasion of important branches of portal veins, hepatic vein, or rarely hepatic artery may sometimes render an operation impossible; however, surgical techniques such as vascular grafting or bridging are sometimes employed to overcome these difficulties.

Tumor Margin

A tumor-free margin of healthy parenchyma of at least 1 cm should be resected with the tumor. Positive resection margins or minimal residual macroscopic disease reduce the median survival of patients with colorectal carcinoma metastases [1]. Tumors closer than 1 cm to the main portal trunk, the vena cava, or the confluence between the hepatic veins and vena cava have a bad prognosis for resection.

Localization of Tumors

The only real contraindication to liver resection is the impossibility of totally resecting the tumor (with the exception of endocrine active tumors where debulging may be helpful). There are situations related to the location of the tumor that render surgery virtually impossible; for example, tumors infiltrating the venous confluence are rarely resectable. Manifestation in multiple segments cranial and caudal to the transverse plane in both lobes and multifocal manifestation render tumors nonresectable.

Because of grim prognosis, the presence of extrahepatic metastasis, even if resected, should probably preclude liver resection [2]. As an exception, surgery for hepatic and pulmonary metastases of colorectal cancer has been undertaken with a curative intent in a growing percentage of cases in recent years. Presence

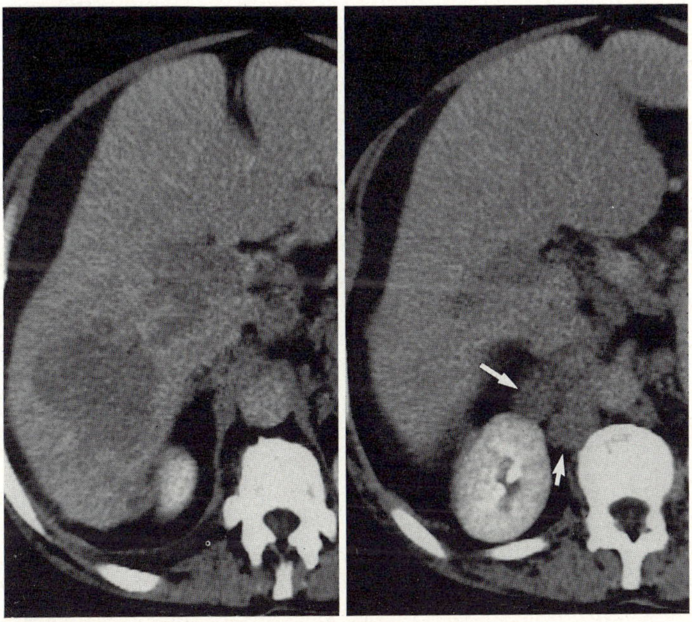

Fig. 4.1. Inoperable hepatocellular carcinoma in patient with alcoholic liver cirrhosis. Note presence of adenopathy (*arrows*)

of positive perihepatic lymphadenopathy is also considered a contraindication to surgery (Fig. 4.1). Surgical contraindications are the following:

Intrahepatic localization: multiple, multifocal, below and above the transverse plane of the liver

Vessels: infiltration of the vena cava, portal vein, or confluence of vena cava and hepatic veins

Metastases: distant metastases (with exception of pulmonary metastases of colorectal cancer); peritoneal seeding

Adenopathy: positive perihepatic or retroperitoneal lymphadenopathy

Cirrhosis: Relative contraindication—depends on stage of cirrhosis and size of resection

Cirrhosis

Cirrhosis is considered by most surgeons to be a contraindication to major resection. A cirrhotic liver lacks the regeneration capacity of normal liver. The greater the extent of resection the more dangerous the procedure is as patients are at risk of hepatic failure.

The introduction, mainly in Japan, of mass screening of patients at risk of hepatocellular carcinomas has improved the early detection of smaller tumors. This leads to an increased resectability of the tumors while the extent of resection remains limited.

Various tests such as Bromsulphalein excretion, indocyanine green clearance, and protein level below 3 g/l can help in selecting cirrhotic patients with sufficient hepatic reserve to undergo resection surgery.

In 1964 Child and Turcotte [3] introduced a grading system to assess the risk of surgery in patients with liver disease (Table 4.1). This classification system, although crude, has served surprisingly well. The main problem is that patients fulfilling all the criteria for grade A or C are rare, and therefore most patients are graded B. Various modifications of Child and Turcotte's original

Table 4.1. Child and Turcotte's classification for estimation of hepatic reserve

Criteria	Grade A	Grade B	Grade C
Serum bilirubin (mg/100 ml)	<2.4	<2.3–2.9	>2.9
Serum albumin (g/100 ml)	>3.5	3.0–3.5	<3.0
Ascites	None	Easily controlled	Poorly controlled
Encephalopathy	None	Minimal	Coma
Nutrition	Good	Moderate	Poor, wasting

Table 4.2. Pugh's modification of Child and Turcotte's grading system

Criteria	1 point	2 point	3 point
Bilirubin (mg/100 ml)	<1–2	2–3	>3
Bilirubin (mg/100 ml) for primary biliary cirrhosis	<1–4	4–10	>10
Albumin (g/l)	>35	28–35	<28
Ascites	Absent	Slight	Moderate
Encephalopathy[a]	None	1 and 2	3 and 4
Prothrombin (s prolonged)	1–4	4–6	>6

[a]According to grading of Trey et al. [40]. Grade A = 5–6 points. grade B = 7–9 points. grade C = 10–15 points.

Table 4.3. Okuda's staging of primary liver cancer

Tumor size	>50% of liver +	<50% of liver −
Ascites	Present +	Absent −
Serum albumin (g/100 ml)	<3.0 +	>3.0 −
Serum bilirubin (mg/100 ml)	>3.0 +	<3.0 −

Stage I = 4 (−): stage II = 1 or 2 (+); stage III = 3 or 4 (+).

grading have been proposed; the most widely used is that of Pugh et al. [4] which omits the assessment of nutrition but introduces the prolongation of prothrombine time (Table 4.2). Grade C is generally considered to be a major contraindication to resection surgery. Okuda et al. [5] introduced a staging scheme taking in account tumor size and liver function, and this is now widely in use in the literature on treating hepatocellular carcinoma (Table 4.3). Depending on the type and location of the lesions, different techniques such as tumorectomy, segmentectomy, or hepatectomy are employed. These are discussed below.

4.1.2 Tumorectomy

Tumorectomy or wedge resection is the least invasive of the resection techniques and is reserved for small, superficial, and isolated lesions. A 1-cm margin of healthy parenchyma should be resected with the tumor. Tumorectomy is often performed during the operation for resection of the primary colorectal carcinoma.

4.1.3 Segmentectomy and Hepatectomy

Segmentectomy is an intermediate step between tumorectomy and major hepatic resections. It involves resection of one or more liver segments. Commonly resected segments are IV (quadrate lobe), V, and VI. Plurisegmentectomy of segments IV, V, and VI or a variation called transverse hepatectomy consisting of en bloc resection of segments IVb, V, and VI are also possible. Resection of segment IV is useful as treatment of lesions lying only in the quadrate lobe. Resection for infiltrating gallbladder cancer generally requires resection of segments IV, V, and sometimes VI, as the gallbladder lies in the fossa between segments IV and V. Segmentectomies conserve liver parenchyma and thus are especially useful in patients with liver cirrhosis. Various possibilities of liver resection are shown in Fig. 4.2.

In partial hepatectomies there are essentially four types of major resection. Depending on the classification in use [41, 42], the terminology varies (see Table 4.4 and Fig. 4.2).

Major liver resection consists essentially of mobilizing hepatic tissue and isolating the vessels supplying the areas to be removed. Technically, this can be carried out either by dissecting the portal pedicle and vessels outside the liver or by searching for the vessels deep in the liver parenchyma after division of the liver, using an ultrasonic dissector or a suction dissector. A combination of techniques is often used. Ex situ resection of the liver is a new experimental surgical technique allowing liver tumors otherwise regarded as irresectable to be removed [6]. With this technique, the liver is freed from its attachments and is taken out of the body. The cancer is removed from the explanted organ, which is then reimplanted.

4.1.4 Results and Factors Influencing Survival

There are very few studies of liver cancer prospectively comparing the survival of patients treated or not treated by liver resection. In most articles, survival of

Table 4.4. Types of hepatectomy

Couinaud 1957 [41]	Goldsmith and Woodburn 1957 [42]	Segments
Right hepatectomy	Right hepatic lobectomy	V, VI, VII, VIII
Left hepatectomy	Left hepatic lobectomy	II, III, IV, perhaps I
Right lobectomy	Extended right lobectomy	IV, V, VI, VII, VIII, perhaps I
Left lobectomy	Left lateral segmentectomy	II, III
Extended left hepatectomy	Extended left lobectomy	II, III, IV, V, VIII

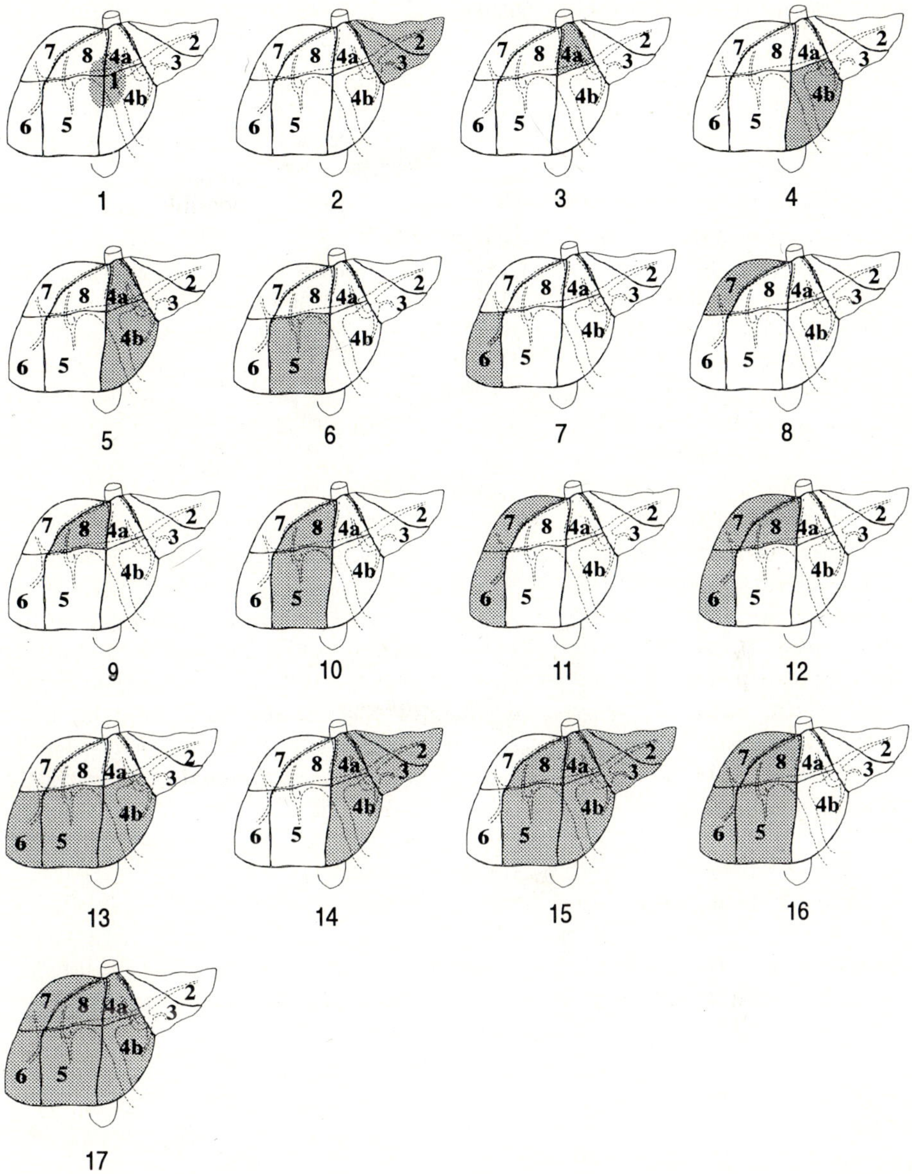

Fig. 4.2. Hepatic resections. *1*, Segment 1 (caudate lobe); *2*, segments 2 and 3; *3*, hemisegment 4a; *4*, hemisegment 4b; *5*, segment 4 (quadrate lobe); *6*, segment 5; *7*, segment 6; *8*, segment 7; *9*, segment 8; *10*, segments 5 and 8; *11*, segments 6 and 7; *12*, segments 6, 7, and 8; *13*, segments 5, 6 and hemisegment 4b (transverse hepatectomy); *14*, segments 2, 3, and 4 (anatomic left liver); *15*, segments 2, 3, 4, 5, and 8 (extended left liver); *16*, segments 5, 6, 7, and 8 (anatomic right liver); *17*, segments 1, 4, 5, 6, 7, and 8 (extended right liver)

operated patients is compared with historical studies on the natural history of the disease. Defining the natural history of liver cancer is not an easy task. Availability of health care facilities, quality of follow-up, and imaging modalities may influence the survival curve. Today the presence of neoplastic lesions in the liver is probably perceived earlier thanks to the greater availability and improved performance of diagnostic modalities. This earlier recognition results in survival times seeming longer, a bias that should be considered when analyzing data comparing survival of patients receiving any kind of treatment with historical survival curves of nontreated patients. Nevertheless, it is now established that untreated patients rarely achieve a 5-year survival, whereas several reports in the literature show that hepatic surgery may provide a 5-year survival about 10%–45%. Benefits of surgery after 2–3 years are not easy to assess as a significant proportion of non-treated patients may survive this period of time.

Hepatocellular Carcinoma

For patients with hepatocellular carcinoma, surgical resection or liver transplantation represents the only hope of cure; unfortunately, however, only a few patients can be operated on. Resectability rates are difficult to assess as most reports take into account only patients presented to the surgeons for operative decision. Frequently, however, hepatocellular carcinomas are discovered without surgical consultation by radiologists or primary physicians and are considered to be nonresectable because they have already grown beyond the limits of resection. Resectability rates of hepatocellular carcinomas in non-cirrhotic patients in Western countries is as low as 10%–28%, and would probably be lower if all patients, even those primarily considered to be inoperable by nonsurgeons, were taken into account.

The presence and type of cirrhosis influences the outcome of surgery and explains differences in experiences between Eastern and Western surgeons. In the East, cirrhosis is most often posthepatitic, whereas in Western countries cirrhosis is more often alcohol related. In the East, however, because of more intensive screening of risk population, the resected tumors tend to be smaller, correlating with a higher resectability rate in cirrhotic patients. Results must be interpreted with respect to these differences. In a Japanese study of 850 patients with hepatocellular carcinoma Okuda et al. [7] reported natural history and prognosis in relation to treatment. Data compiled from this large study are shown in Table 4.5. Results and survival in various international series are listed in Table 4.6.

Recurrence of Tumor

In a study [10] of 123 patients surveyed after hepatectomy for small hepatocellular carcinoma (<5 cm), 54.2% of patients had tumor recurrence in the residual liver (Fig. 4.3). Survival of different subgroups and the effect of

Table 4.5. Survival of 850 patients with hepatocellular carcinoma in terms of Okuda's staging system and type of treatment

	Stage I		Stage II		Stage III	
	n	Median survival (months)	*n*	Median survival (months)	*n*	Median survival (months)
Entire group	272	11.5	466	3.0	112	0.9
No treatment	33	8.3	134	2.0	62	0.7
Surgery	115	25.6	42	12.2		
Surgery tumor < 25%	88	29.0				
Surgery tumor > 25% – <50%	27	8.1				
Medical treatment	124	9.4	290	3.6	50	1.6
Embolization	41	10.4	64	9.5		
Chemoembolization						
Arterial chemotherapy	55	10.3	141	3.7	26	1.3
Systemic chemotherapy	23	4.3	82	2.5	17	1.4

Table 4.6. Results of resection surgery of hepatocellular carcinoma

Country	*n*	Size	Survival 1 year %	Survival 3 year %	Survival 5 year %	Mortality %	Reference
Japan	123	<5 cm	84	42	19	4	[8]
Japan	809	various	56	31	—	—	[7]
France	35	various	66	33	—	14	[9]

chemoembolization is presented in Table 4.7. It is interesting that chemoembolization had an effect on short-time survival as more patients survived 1 year than in the group with no treatment. In the group treated by chemoembolization, there were also long-term survivors, absent in the untreated group.

Metastases to the Liver of Colorectal Carcinoma

In a large series of 1209 patients with colorectal liver metastases, Scheele et al. [1] showed that radical excision of colorectal metastases to the liver offers an effective palliation and probably a chance of cure in a small group of patients. Patients who underwent hepatic resection with curative intent demonstrated a prolonged survival time by a median of 1 year compared to the groups of nonradically resected or untreated patients. Untreated patients and patients with nonresectable lesions failed to achieve 5-year survival. Among 183 patients with potentially curative surgery 173 were alive after the operation (5.5% mortality), 25 after 5 years, and 7 after 10 years. The influence of different factors on survival is shown in Table 4.8.

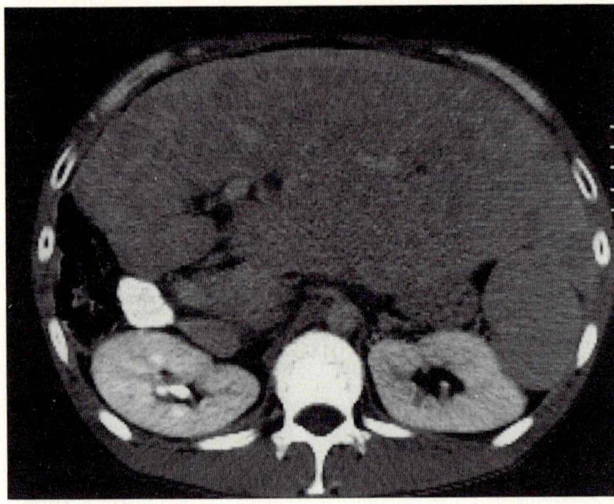

Fig. 4.3. Diffuse nodular recurrence of hepatocellular carcinoma in residual liver 4 months after resection of right liver

Table 4.7. Survival of 123 patients after hepatectomy for small (<5 cm) hepatocellular carcinoma. Data compiled from [10]

	1-year survival %	3-year survival %	5-year survival %
All patients	84.2	42.7	19.1
Patients without recurrence	—	—	48.9
All patients with recurrence	—	—	11.0
Patients with recurrence and chemoembolization treatment	70.3	45.0	14.9
Patients with recurrence and without chemoembolization treatment	37.1	0.0	0.0

In a prospective randomized study evaluating various treatment modalities of colorectal cancer metastatic to the liver it was shown that median survival correlated with the extent of the disease [12]. In the group of patients with solitary resectable metastases, adjunction of continuous hepatic artery infusion of fluorodeoxyuridine to resection did not change survival. In the group of patients with multiple resectable metastases there was no benefit of surgery in terms of survival when comparing patients who underwent surgery and continuous hepatic artery infusion with those who had continuous hepatic artery

Table 4.8. Factors influencing survival of patients with colorectal metastases to the liver (data compiled from [11])

	5-year survival %
Extrahepatic disease	
No extrahepatic disease	32
Extrahepatic disease (lung, adrenals, peritoneum)	20
Portal, celiac nodes	4
Tumor-free margin of liver resection	44
> 10 mm	
< 10 mm	26
Positive margin	18
Number of metastases	
1	37
2	34
3	9
4 or more	18

infusion only. Repeated resections have been performed with success, with an operative mortality rate of 5.2% [13].

Patterns of recurrence following hepatic resection for metastases of colorectal cancer are of interest. In a large multi-institutional study of 607 patients who had undergone resection of isolated hepatic metastases with curative intent [14], 5-year disease-free survival was of 25%. At the time of the report 70% of patients had recurrences: 43% of patients had recurrences in the liver, 31% of the patients developed lung metastases, and 13% had locoregional recurrence at the site of resection of the primary tumor. The rate of peritoneal recurrences is difficult to assess, as this type of recurrence is seldom recognized by imaging techniques.

In a study of 100 long-term survivors (over 5 years), it appears that patients with a small number of metastases and localized primary disease have a survival advantage. Interestingly, long-term survivors in the poor-prognosis subgroup were found: one patient with positive resection margin, three with bilobar metastases, 30 with stage C cancer, and 12 with metastases greater than 8 cm [15].

Summary

Patients surviving 5 years after the detection of liver metastases without resection are extremely rare, whereas 5-year survival after resection is commonly found in more than 25% of patients. The operative mortality of about 5% is acceptable for patients who have no alternative treatment. Resection is recommended in all patients in whom resection with curative intent is possible. A 1-cm tumor-free resection margin should be obtained whenever possible.

The only absolute contraindication of resection surgery is the impossibility of radical tumor removal. Surgery should not be performed if residual disease remains. The presence of perihepatic adenopathy should also be considered a contraindication because of very poor prognosis.

Metastases to the Liver of Noncolorectal Neoplasms

The largest accumulated experience with hepatic resection for metastases is with cancers of colorectal origin. Experience with resection for metastases of noncolorectal origin is small, mainly because metastases localized to a resectable area of the liver are unusual [16], and because extrahepatic spread is often encountered. Reports in literature are sparse [17] ; however, resections of liver metastases from a variety of primary cancers have been performed. Operative mortality (3%–5%) is about the same as in resection for metastases of colorectal origin. Resection of metastases of neuroendocrine tumors, even when incomplete, may be of interest. Volume diminution of the often slowly growing tumors may reduce the potential lethal hormonal activity of these tumors and offer an effective palliation.

Cholangiocarcinoma

Cholangiocarcinoma, a tumor derived from the bile duct epithelium, occurs less frequently than hepatocellular carcinoma or liver metastases. Surgical experience is also smaller. Cholangiocarcinoma may be separated into peripheral, arising from small bile ducts within the liver, and hilar, arising from the major hepatic ducts near or at the junction (Klatskin's tumors) of right and left hepatic ducts. Prognosis is poor, and patients generally die of sepsis or hepatic failure. Median survival of nonresectable patients is 3–6 months. Surgical management of both peripheral and hilar cholangiocarcinoma consists of major hepatic resection generally combined with cholangioenteric anastomoses. Curative resection is possible in about 10%–25% of patients. Median survival is about 1.5 years [18]; 5-year survivors are rare [19].

4.1.5 Complications of Resection Surgery

Previously reported mortality rates of up to 20%, largely due to bleeding, liver failure, and infection, have been drastically decreased by improvements of surgical technique and increasing experience. Mortality rates of hepatic resection are now 0%–5.5% for colorectal metastases and 10%–15% for hepatocellular carcinomas.

Table 4.9. Most frequently reported complications of hepatic resection for all indications

	Frequency approximate %
Pulmonary	
Pneumonia	~20
Pleural effusion	~10–15
Gastrointestinal	
Subphrenic abscess	~5–10
Infection	~20
Bile leak	~5–10
Hepatic failure	~4–8
Diverse	
Cardiac failure	~3–6
Wound infection	~5–10

In a painstaking report of all complications [20], moderate and severe complications were found in 35%, mild complications in 24% and no complications in 38% of patients having undergone hepatic resection for metastatic colorectal carcinoma. In this series mean anesthesia time was of 448 min and mean estimated blood loss of 3663 ml. Mean hospital stay was 17.5 days (range 8–52 days). A list of complication most frequently reported in literature is found in Table 4.9.

4.2 Arterial Ligature: Dearterialization

Normal liver parenchyma obtains about 75% of its blood supply from the portal veins and 25% from the hepatic arteries whereas in cirrhotic livers the blood supply is obtained from the arteries in a proportion up to 75%. Very small liver tumors (smaller than 5 mm) are fed mainly by portal veins; becoming larger, these lesions receive up to 95% of their blood supply from hepatic arteries. For a very long time surgeons believed that ligation of the hepatic arteries is nearly always fatal. It was not until it was proven that bacterial overgrowth was the cause of deaths occurring after ligation of the hepatic artery that this technique was investigated as possible treatment for hepatic tumors. Although some successes were noted in experimental studies on liver tumors in rats, results were disappointing in man. After ligation of the hepatic artery, collaterals develop almost immediately from capsular branches or the phrenic arteries. The development of these collaterals takes place within a few days. Intrahepatic collaterals may develop within minutes, a fact well known to interventional angiographers. Further, it is now known that the decrease in blood flow by 90% to liver metastases after hepatic artery ligation is not sufficient to achieve a complete cure since the portal blood supply always spares a rim of neoplastic cells around the necrotic area.

After hepatic dearterialization transaminases increase steadily within the first 24–48 h and indicate parenchymal destruction. Lysosomal enzymes are released from the ischemic parenchyma. Liver function is altered: the synthesis of proteins is transiently reduced, levels of coagulation factors drop, and bile production decreases. There is also a rapid depletion of glycogen, and glycolysis is stimulated.

Cytotoxic oxygen-derived free radicals are also involved in liver ischemia and are produced early after interruption of the hepatic arterial flow with no obvious increase after reperfusion [21].

In tumors, the vessels and especially the endothelium are most sensitive to hypoxia [22]. Tumor cells themselves show varying sensitivity to hypoxia; some depend more on aerobic glucose utilization whereas others are dependent on anaerobic metabolism.

4.2.1 Techniques

Hepatic dearterialization consists of ligation of the hepatic artery close to the liver. Structures in the hepatoduodenal ligament are dissected, and all ligamentous attachments of the liver are disconnected.

In repeated transient hepatic dearterialization all ligamentous attachments of the liver are disconnected, and the hepatic artery is surrounded by an occluding sling or vascular occluder. With this technique the repeated transient ischemic periods may be delayed postoperatively, sparing healthy liver tissue.

4.2.2 Results

No randomized study has shown any benefit in long-term survival of patients with hepatocellular carcinomas or nonendocrine liver metastases treated by hepatic artery ligation, dearterialization, or repeated transient hepatic dearterialization. Tumor response was reported in 8 of 13 patients (2 patients with hepatocellular carcinomas and 11 with liver metastases of colorectal origin) treated by a combination of dearterialization and intraperitoneal chemotherapy [23]. Results of some studies are listed in Table 4.10. Better results are obtained in treatment of patients with carcinoid tumors metastatic to the liver, although no improvements over other methods of treatment have been shown.

Overall dearterialization techniques have not proven their value. Results obtained in combination with chemotherapy are comparable to those obtained with chemotherapy alone. Besides noticeable mortality rates, the technique is hampered by high complication rates. Further, as a major inconvenience, interventional catheter techniques (embolization, chemoembolization, etc.) become nearly impossible after hepatic artery ligation.

Table 4.10. Results of dearterialization procedures

Type of tumor	*n*	Occlusion	Chemotherapy	Survival (months)	Mortality (%)	Reference
Hepatocellular carcinomas	37	—	—	1.9(med.)	27(at 1 mo.)	[24]
	33	Dearterialization	—	1.1(med.)	44(at 1 mo.)	
	30	HAL	5-FU ia +DOX	1.1(med.)	42(at 1 mo.)	
	29	HAL	5-FU ip +DOX	2.7(med.)	32(at 1 mo.)	
	37	Radiation	—	2.2(med.)	15(at 1 mo.)	
Metastases of colorectal carcinoma	21	Temporary dearterialization	5-FU ia	11.2(mean)	10	[25]
	23	—	5-FU ia	11.5(mean)	0	
Metastases of colorectal carcinoma	20	HAL	5-FU ip	11(mean)		[26]
	20	—	—	11(mean)		

HAL, Hepatic artery ligation; DOX, doxorubicin; *ip* intraperitoneal; *ia*, intraarterial; *med*, median, *mo*, month.

4.3 Cryosurgery

Cryosurgery is a technique for destroying tumors by cold. Most cells undergo internal freezing at temperatures under −20°C and die either immediately or during the subsequent thawing. Using two or more freeze-thawing cycles may increase the likelihood of cell necrosis. Obliteration of small blood vessels contributes to hypoxic cell death.

After a right subcostal incision the liver is exposed. Lesions are localized intraoperatively with ultrasound. A probe, in which liquid nitrogen at −196°C circulates, is introduced into the center of the tumor. Besides detection of the lesions, ultrasound is used to guide the positioning of the probe and to monitor the freeze-thawing cycles. As the extent of necrosis can be predicted, it is important to include within the frozen area a small rim of healthy liver parenchyma around the tumor.

Cryosurgery is not tissue specific, and various types of tumors can be treated. Encouraging results have been obtained in hepatocellular carcinomas smaller than 5 cm in diameter, with a 5-year survival rate of 37.5% [27]. Healthy liver tissue can be spared, and cryosurgery can thus be an effective alternative to liver resection in patients with low hepatic functional reserve [28]. Complications are infrequent; however, a near-fatal nitrogen embolism has recently been described [29]. In principle this technique could be compared to percutaneous alcoholization of liver tumors, a technique that also spares healthy liver tissue, treats neoplastic tissues focally, and has comparable short- and long-term results (see Chap. 6). The advantage of cryosurgery is the use of intraoperative ultrasound, a very sensitive technique that allows detection of previous unnoticed metastases, the disadvantage being the need for laparotomy. In the future this advantage will probably be compensated by improvements in imaging techniques such as MR.

4.4 Transplantation

Liver transplantation has emerged from the experimental stage. Widespread increase of liver transplantation worldwide is due to improved immunosuppressive drugs and better defined treatment protocols. Survival rates of patients after transplantation have improved and depend on the underlying disease leading to transplantation and the stage of the disease. Classical indications for liver transplantation include [30, 31]:

- Primary biliary cirrhosis
- Inactive alcoholic cirrhosis
- Chronic active hepatitis
- Fulminant/subfulminant hepatic necrosis
- Sclerosing cholangitis
- Primary hepatic neoplasms
- Budd-Chiari syndrome
- Metabolic diseases
- Biliary atresia
- Polycystic disease

In malignant disease transplantation is performed when cancer is considered to be nonresectable, or when repeated resections have failed [13].

There is no substantial consensus about whether a liver transplantation is justified for the treatment of hepatic malignancies. Because of disease recurrence, the results of liver transplantation for metastatic liver disease have not been as favorable as for other indications such as end-stage cirrhosis. In a retrospective study of disease recurrence after transplantation for various indications in 106 patients, recurrence of hepatocellular carcinoma was found in 46% of the patients and hepatitis B recurred in 79% [32]. When transplantation is performed for malignancy, noncirrhotic patients with hepatocellular carcinoma, especially the fibrolamellar subtype, have the best prognosis whereas cholangiocarcinoma and large hepatocellular carcinoma in cirrhotic patients and metastases have the worst prognosis and the highest recurrence rates [33, 34]. Small hepatocellular carcinomas associated with cirrhosis are also considered a valuable indication for transplantation as resection surgery on patients with cirrhosis is problematic.

Liver metastases are generally not considered a good indication for transplantation; however, the unique group of neuroendocrine tumors is an exception as their slow growth allows liver transplantation effectively to palliate and control symptoms [35]. Careful preoperative patient selection based on liver biopsy, CT of the thorax and the abdomen, pre-transplant laparotomy, and restriction of transplantation to lymph node negative patients seems to improve survival and opens the concept of tumor growth enhancement by immunosuppresive to question [36]. Contraindications to liver transplantation are as follows:

Absolute contraindications
- Extrahepatic malignancy
- Advanced sepsis
- Advanced cardiopulmonary disease
- Active drug or alcohol abuse
- Multiple noncorrectable congenital anomalies

Relative contraindications
- Age >60 years
- Irreversible renal failure
- Prior extensive biliary surgery
- Portal vein thrombosis
- HBsAg positivity
- Major psychosocial disorders
- HIV positivity

In patients with liver malignancies 5-year survival rates of 30%–39% have been achieved with liver transplantation, mostly in the subgroup of patients with small hepatocellular carcinoma (<5 cm). Careful patient selection is of the utmost importance. Transplantation for malignancy should be reserved for patients considered to be inoperable for resection surgery with no extrahepatic spread and negative lymph node staging. Selection of the type of tumor is also important; metastases, sarcoma, and cholangiocarcinoma are considered as the worst indication [38].

The scarcity of available donor organs precludes widespread use of transplantation in patients with liver cancer. In the competition for the sparse donor organs, patients with benign end-stage diseases should be favored. A better harvesting organization, international collaboration, and restriction of the number of centers for performing transplantation are problems to be resolved [39].

References

1. Scheele J, Stangl R, Altendorf-Hofmann A (1990) Hepatic metastases from colorectal carcinoma: impact of surgical resection on the natural history. Br J Surg 77: 1241–1246
2. Foster JH (1990) Surgical treatment of metastatic liver tumors. Hepatogastroenterology 37(2): 182–187
3. Child CG III, Turcotte JG (1964) Surgery and portal hypertension. In: Child CG III (ed) The liver and portal hypertension. Saunders, Philadelphia; p 50
4. Pugh RNH, Murray-Lyon IM, Dawson JL, Pietroni MC, Williams R (1973) Transection of the oesophagus for bleeding oesophageal varices. Br J Surg 60: 646–649

5. Okuda K, Obata H, Nakajima Y, Ohtsuki T, Okazaki N, Ohnishi K (1984) Prognosis of primary hepatocellular carcinoma. Hepatology 4: 3S–6S
6. Pichlmayr R, Grosse H, Hauss J, Gubernatis G, Lamesch P, Bretschneider HJ (1990) Technique and preliminary results of extracorporeal liver surgery (bench procedure) and of surgery on the in situ perfused liver. Br J Surg 77(1): 21–26
7. Okuda K, Ohtsuki T, Obata H, Tomimatsu M, Okazaki N, Hasegawa H, Nakajima Y, Ohnishi K (1985) Natural history of hepatocellular carcinoma and prognosis in relation to treatment. Study of 850 patients. Cancer 56: 918–928
8. Lai EC, Choi TK, Tong SW, Ong GB, Wong J (1986) Treatment of unresectable hepatocellular carcinoma: results of a randomized controlled trial. World J Surg 10: 501–509
9. Bismuth H, Houssin D, Ornowski J, Meriggi F (1986) Liver resections in cirrhotic patients: a Western experience. World J Surg 10: 311–317
10. Takayasu K, Muramatsu Y, Moriyama N, Hasegawa H, Makuuchi M, Okazaki N, Hirohashi S, Tsugane S (1989) Clinical and radiologic assessments of the results of hepatectomy for small hepatocellular carcinoma and therapeutic arterial embolization for postoperative recurrence. Cancer 64: 1848–1852
11. Hughes K, Scheele J, Sugarbaker PH (1989) Surgery for colorectal cancer metastatic to the liver. Optimizing the results of treatment. Surg Clin North Am 69: 339–359
12. Wagman LD, Kemeny MM, Leong L, Terz JJ, Hill LR, Beatty JD, Kokal WA, Riihimaki DU (1990) A prospective, randomized evaluation of the treatment of colorectal cancer metastatic to the liver. J Clin Oncol 8(11): 1885–1893
13. Huguet C, Bona S, Nordlinger B, Lagrange L, Parc R, Harb J, Benard F (1990) Repeat hepatic resection for primary and metastatic carcinoma of the liver. Surg Gynecol Obstet 171(5): 398–402
14. Hughes KS et al. (1986) Resection of the liver for colorectal carcinoma metastases: a multi-institutional study of patterns of recurrence. Surgery 100: 278
15. Hughes KS, Rosenstein RB, Songhorabodi S, Adson MA, Ilstrup DM, Fortner JG, Maclean BJ, Foster JH, Daly JM, Fitzherbert D et al. (1988) Resection of the liver for colorectal carcinoma metastases. A multi-institutional study of long-term survivors. Dis Colon Rectum 31: 1–4
16. Blumgart LH (1987) Hepatic resection for tumor. Ther Umsch 4: 456–463
17. Nudelmann LI, Cabot R, Benjamin IS, Blumgart LH (1989) Hepatic resection for secondary tumours. Cancer Surv 8(1): 33–48
18. Burcharth F (1988) Klatskin tumours. Acta Chir Scand Suppl 541: 63–69
19. Chen MF, Jan YY, Wang CS, Jeng LB, Hwang TL (1989) Clinical experience in 20 hepatic resections for peripheral cholangiocarcinoma. Cancer 64: 2226–2232
20. Vetto JT, Hughes KS, Rosenstein R, Sugarbaker PH (1990) Morbidity and mortality of hepatic resection for metastatic colorectal carcinoma. Dis Colon Rectum 33: 408–413
21. Puntis MCA, Peerson BG, Jönsson G et al. (1987) Free radical production in the ischemic rat liver. Surg Res Commun 1: 17
22. Denekamp J (1984) Vascular endothelium as the vulnerable element in tumors. Acta Radiol [Oncol] 23: 217
23. Persson BG, Jeppsson B, Ekberg H, Tranberg KG, Lundstedt C, Bengmark S (1990) Repeated dearterialization of hepatic tumors with an implantable occluder. Cancer 66: 1139–1146
24. Lai EC, Choi TK, Tong SW, Ong GB, Wong J (1986) Treatment of unresectable hepatocellular carcinoma: results of a randomized controlled trial. World Surg 10: 501–509
25. Ekberg H, Tranberg KG, Lundstedt C, Hanff G, Ranstam J, Jeppsson B, Bengmark S (1986) Determinants of survival after intraarterial infusion of 5-fluorouracil for liver metastases from colorectal cancer: a multivariate analysis. J Surg Oncol 31: 246–254
26. Gerard A, Dalesio O, Duez N, Lise M, Pector JC, Bleiberg H, Nitti D, Willems G, Delvaux G (1986) Hepatic arterial ligation and portal vein infusion: a clinical trial by the Gastrointestinal Tract Cancer Group of the European Organization for Research and Treatment of Cancer. Recent Results Cancer Res 100: 276–281
27. Zhou XD, Tang ZY, Yu YQ, Ma ZC (1988) Clinical evaluation of cryosurgery in the treatment of primary liver cancer. Report of 60 cases. Cancer 61: 1889–1892

28. Ravikumar TS, Steele GD (1989) Hepatic cryosurgery. Clin North Am 69: 433–440
29. Schlinkert RT, Chapman TP (1990) Nitrogen embolus as a complication of hepatic cryosurgery. Arch Surg 125: 1214
30. Naouri A, Tissot E (1990) Indications de la transplantation hépatique chez l'adulte. J Chir (Paris) 127(6–7): 334–340
31. Pouyet M, Ducerf C, Gaussorgues P, Salord F, Sirodot M, Caillon P, Dubois JM, Rivoire M, Baulieux J, Bouletreau P et al. (1989) Hépatites fulminantes et sub-fulminantes traitées par transplantation orthotopique du foie. A propos de dix cas. Chirurgie 115(8): 533–539
32. Hart J, Busutti RW, Lewin KJ (1990) Disease recurrence following liver transplantation. Am J Surg Pathol 14 Suppl 1: 79–91
33. Olthoff KM, Millis JM, Rosove MH, Goldstein LI, Ramming KP, Busuttil RW (1990) Is liver transplantation justified for the treatment of hepatic malignancies? Arch Surg 125(8): 1261–1266
34. Ismail T, Angrisani L, Gunson BK, Hubscher SG, Buckels JA, Neuberger JM, Elias E, McMaster P (1990) Primary hepatic malignancy: the role of liver transplantation. Br J Surg 77(9): 983–987
35. Alsina AE, Bartus S, Hull D, Rosson R, Schweizer RT (1990) Liver transplant for metastatic neuroendocrine tumor. J Clin Gastroenterol 12(5): 533–537
36. Lim SM, Pollard SG (1990) Liver transplantation in cancer—a review. Ann Acad Med Singapore 19(2): 275–280
37. Jenkins RL, Fairchild RB (1989) The role of transplantation in liver disease. Surg Clin North Am 69: 371–382
38. Steffen R, Neuhaus P, Blumhardt G, Bechstein WO (1991) Liver transplantation for liver cancer. Onkologie 14: 100–106
39. Rohner A (1990) La transplantation hépatique en Suisse. Premiers résultats. Schweiz Med Wochenschr 120: 563–655
40. Trey C, Burns DG, Saunders SJ (1966) Treatment of hepatic coma by exchange blood transfusion. N Engl J Med 274: 473–481
41. Couinaud C (1957) Le foie. Etudes anatomiques et chirurgicales. Masson, Paris
42. Goldsmith NA, Woodburne RT (1957) The surgical anatomy pertaining to liver resection. Surg Gynecol Obstet 105: 310–318

5 Radiotherapy

5.1 Tolerance of the Liver to Radiation

The liver is a relatively radiosensitive organ. The radiation sensitivity of the liver is to a great extent related to radiation damage of small blood vessels in the liver. Biopsies performed within 2 months after irradiation to dose levels between 30–60 Gy show sinusoidal congestion, hyperemia, loss of central hepatic cells, and vascular changes including loss of endothelium and thickening of intima. Two to four months after irradiation, obliterative changes in efferent veins with collagenous tissue in the lumen are found. After 4 months the specimens reveal fatty vacuolization, vascular changes, centrilobular fibrosis, and atrophy.

Hepatocytes are relatively resistant to radiation and large doses of irradiation are required to cause direct inflammatory changes in the liver. One of the reasons for hepatocyte resistance to radiation is the low mitosis rate. Hepatocytes are long-living cells and divide irregularly and rarely. After cell loss they regenerate rapidly.

Usually the period during and immediately after liver irradiation is clinically silent. It is not until 2–6 weeks after completion of the irradiation that damage to healthy liver parenchyma becomes evident. In radiation hepatitis the liver enlarges, ascites is present, and liver chemistry becomes pathological with elevation of alkaline phosphatase. In favorable cases ascites decreases, and liver chemistry reaches normal values after a few weeks. Radiation hepatitis is seldom encountered when the daily radiation dose does not exceed 2.0 Gy (10 Gy/week) and the total dose does not exceed 30 Gy (Table 5.1). Doses up to 46–50 Gy in 4–5 weeks can be tolerated if only parts of the liver are irradiated. Because of its great regenerative capacity, liver failure should not occur when at least 25% of the organ is shielded.

5.2 External Radiotherapy

Generally, high-energy accelerators (15–25 MeV) are used for irradiation of the liver. Thinner patients can be treated with lower energy. Hepatic irradiation is generally delivered to opposed anterior and posterior fields. For a dose higher than 15 Gy the right kidney should be shielded. Ultrasound or CT are most

Table 5.1. Relationship between delivered tumor dose and radiation hepatitis (compiled from [1])

Gy	*n*	Radiation hepatitis
13–26	5	0
30–34	8	1
34–37	6	2
38–41	18	6
42–51	3	2
Total	40	11

useful for exact location of the liver. CT is also especially useful for dosimetry and planification.

5.2.1 Irradiation with Curative Intention

Because of the low dose of irradiation tolerated by the liver, the best results are obtained in radiosensitive tumors such as ovarian carcinoma, lymphomas, and seminomas. Abdomen irradiation comprising the liver is performed to treat and prevent peritoneal seeding of ovarian carcinoma. After hystero-salpingectomy, 5-year survival increases after whole-abdomen irradiation compared to pelvic irradiation alone [2]. Hepatic manifestation of Hodgkin's lymphoma and non-Hodgkin's lymphoma may be treated with 20–30 Gy in addition to chemotherapy. For ovarian carcinomas and lymphomas, radiotherapy is generally combined with chemotherapy. Seminomas metastastic to the liver may be treated with a dose up to 30 Gy.

Although carcinoid tumors are known to be little radiosensitive, good clinical results after liver irradiation have been obtained. Decrease of liver volume, normalization of serum values of hormonoactive substances have been noted. The dose delivered corresponded to 30 Gy.

5.2.2 Irradiation with Palliative Intention

Besides the above-mentioned indications, irradiation is employed palliatively to treat hepatocellular carcinomas and metastases of lung and breast cancer or of colorectal origin. Irradiation of the liver has virtually no incidence on survival. In a study of 69 patients with liver metastases of various origin, median survival, starting at the beginning of the radiotherapy, was of 4 months [3]. Although a time-consuming method, irradiation is considered to be useful for palliation with doses between 20–30 Gy. Reduction of pain is found in 70% of patients and decrease in jaundice in 28%, anorexia in 77%, and ascites in 50% [4]. In painful livers concentrated irradiations of 2 × 6.5 Gy in 3 days or 3 × 7.5 Gy at 3-week intervals have been proposed [5].

5.2.3 Tolerance to Treatment and Complications

Below doses of 30 Gy irradiation is well supported, but diarrhea, nausea, leukopenia, and thrombocytopenia frequently occur. These side effects are frequently encountered in irradiation of the abdomen.

5.3 Internal Radiotherapy

Due to the radiosensitivity of the liver and the impossibility of applying a sufficient tumor dose by external beam irradiation, various techniques of internal irradiation have been developed. There are four principal ways to apply radiation internally to liver tumors: percutaneous implantation of radioactive seeds such as irridium-192, intraarterial injection of yttrium-90 particles, intraarterial injection of iodine-131 labeled Lipiodol, and intravenous or intraarterial injection of radioactively labeled antibodies.

5.3.1 Percutaneous Implantation of Radioactive Seeds

Percutaneous implantation of radioactive seeds is used mainly for internal radiotherapy of cholangiocarcinomas. The technique consists in catheterizing the biliary tree during percutaneous transhepatic cholangiography. A cannula is placed at the location of the tumor, and the radioactive seeds are then loaded within it and left in place until an adequate dose of radiation is reached locally. The cannula can be exchanged for a drainage tube. Irridium-192 loaded needles have also been placed percutaneously into the center of tumors under sonographic guidance.

5.3.2 Yttrium-90

Yttrium-90 has interesting properties for internal radiation through embolization of ^{90}Y-loaded microspheres. It is a pure β-emitter with a mean tissue penetration of 2.5 mm (maximum 10.3 mm). The mean energy of the β particles is 0.93 MeV (maximum 2.27 MeV), and the half-life is 64 h. Stable ^{89}Y can be activated to radioactive ^{90}Y by neutron bombardment in a nuclear reactor. ^{90}Y-labeled ceramic or resin microspheres have a mean size of 20 μm and have a specific activity of 0.21–0.83 MBq/mg.

The dose can be calculated as [6]:

$$\text{Dose(Gy)} = [\text{activity(Mbq/0.037)} \times 1.822]/\text{weight(in grams)}$$

First trials with ^{90}Y caused deaths from myelosuppression due to unexpected leaching of the yttrium from the surface of the resin microspheres.

Recently, new ^{90}Y glass microspheres have solved the problem of leaching. Prior to injection of the microspheres a ^{99m}Tc microsphere scan is performed to detect extrahepatic shunting and avoid delivering a potential lethal dose of ^{90}Y to the lung. As ^{90}Y is a β-emitter, a relatively high dose can be injected without impairing healthy liver parenchyma. Selectivity of the injection is a problem: the more activity that can be brought about in the tumor and not in healthy parenchyma, the better. Although liver tumors are predominantly fed by arteries, they are not always hypervascular. To overcome this problem vasoconstrictive substance can be injected prior to the injection of ^{90}Y microspheres; tumor vessels have generally lost the ability to constrict, whereas normal vessels show a clear decrease in diameter. Microspheres, however, are directed predominantly to the liver tumor. High doses of radiation can thus be absorbed by the tumor (50–320 Gy).

Several cases of partial response have been described but as yet no cure (Fig. 5.1). Complications using the newer and safer glass microspheres are related mainly to nontarget embolization.

Although the technique for injecting ^{90}Y microspheres is cumbersome and despite the large amount of activity handled during treatments, exposure of the personnel involved is minimal [7].

5.3.3 ^{131}I-Labeled Lipiodol

The avidity of hepatocellular carcinoma for Lipiodol has been employed for internal radiotherapy. ^{131}I-labeled Lipiodol injected intraarterially accumulates in liver tumors. In a study of 15 patients with hepatocellular carcinoma, partial response was found in nine patients, whereas no objective response was seen in the group of patients with metastases [8]. In a study of 50 patients with Okuda stage I or II hepatocellular carcinoma, an objective response was found in 40%. Survival depended significantly on the Okuda stage and on the avidity of the tumor for Lipiodol [9].

Results seem similar to those of other techniques such as chemoembolization; however, randomized controlled studies with direct comparison are required. As it is a cumbersome technique necessitating isolation of patients for radioprotection, it must prove superior to have a future.

5.3.4 Radiolabeled Antibodies

Radiolabeled antibodies may be helpful in detecting undiscovered metastases, but they are of no use yet in treatment as no sufficient activity can be brought to the target [10]. For this reason, ^{131}I-labeled monoclonal antibodies against carcinoembryogenic antigen was administered to two patients using intrametastatic injections resulting in a slowing the tumor growth [11]. Although the perspective may be fascinating, enormous problems remain: creating antibodies

a

b

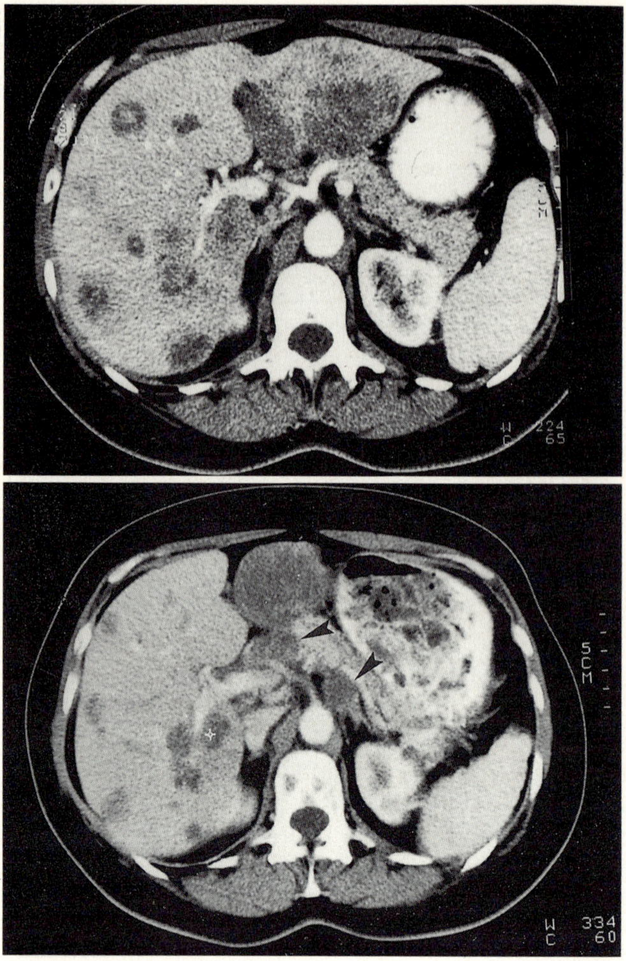

Fig. 5.1. **a** A 52-year old patient with diffuse liver metastases of breast carcinoma. **b** Partial response in same patient 11 months after first and 9 months after second embolization with ^{90}Y resin particles. Note decrease in size and hypodensity of the focal liver lesions. Note also growth of extrahepatic disease in left adrenal and in peripancreatic adenopathy (*arrowheads*). (Courtesy of Prof. Rösler and PD Dr. Becker, Inselspital Bern)

directed specifically against the tumor and with no activity against healthy body tissues in sufficient quantity and bringing sufficient activity to the tumor.

Summary

At present, experience with internal radiotherapy is too small for definite conclusions. Long-term survival cannot be analyzed yet. Brachytherapy with

^{192}Ir seeds is often the only hope for palliation of inoperable patients with cholangiocarcinomas. Intraarterial injection of ^{90}Y or ^{131}I-labeled Lipiodol seem promising methods; these techniques are, however, cumbersome and have not yet proven their value or shown their superiority over selective chemotherapy in large controlled studies.

5.4 Radiotherapy Combined with Chemotherapy

Drugs such as 5-fluorouracil (5-FU) in combination with irradiation enhance cell killing [12] and increase median survival in colorectal cancer [13]. In a sequential nonrandomized study of 48 patients with metastases of colorectal origin, 8 were treated with 5-FU alone, 14 with hepatic irradiation alone, and 25 with a combination of intraarterial 5-FU and irradiation. The median survival of the different groups was 190, 270, and 376 days, respectively [14]. Patients treated with doxorubicin are at higher risk of radiation hepatitis, and the radiation dose should be reduced to 20 Gy. Results of irradiation of hepatic metastases combined with intraarterial chemotherapy are generally not better than those of chemotherapy alone (Table 5.2; see also Chaps. 7, 8). Several trials are now studying the possible role of hepatic radiation as adjuvant therapy in colorectal carcinoma.

In a study of 194 patients with hepatocellular carcinoma, the combination of chemotherapy (intravenous doxorubicin and 5-FU) and radiotherapy produced a response rate of about 20%, hyperfractioning increasing toxicity when compared to standard irradiation [19]. In a series of 28 patients treated by a combination of transcatheter arterial embolization and irradiation 5-year survival was of 27.8%, and the partial response rate was 82.1%. The authors found the combination therapy to be superior to arterial embolization alone [20]. The important difference in response rates of these studies may be explained partially by the fact that transcatheter arterial embolization is known to be more effective on hepatocellular carcinoma than intravenous chemotherapy.

Table 5.2. Combination of radiotherapy and chemotherapy of liver metastases

Drug	Radiation dose	n	Response %	Survival (months)	Reference
5-FU intraarterial	25.5 Gy, 1.5 Gy/day	19	47	6	[15]
FUDR or 5-FU	21 Gy, 14 fractions	12	83	17	[16]
5-FU and methotrexate	30 Gy in 4 weeks	12	25		[17]
5-FU and doxorubicin	13.5, 21 Gy	22	55		[18]

5-FU, Fluorouracil; FUDR, Fluorodeoxyuridine

References

1. Ingold JA, Reed GB, Kaplan HS, Bagshaw MA (1965) Radiation hepatitis. AJR AM J Roentgenol 93: 200–208
2. Bush RS (1983) Radiation therapy for patients with ovarian cancer. Strahlentherapie 159: 131–137
3. Heimdal K, Hannisdal E, Fossa SD (1988) Survival after palliative radiotherapy of liver metastases. A search for prognostic factors. Acta Oncol 27: 63–65
4. Prasad B, Lee MS, Hendrickson FR (1977) Irradiation of hepatic metastases. Int J Radiat Oncol Biol Phys 2: 129–132
5. Vigner H (1985) Radiothérapie des cancers secondaires du foie. Ann Gastroenterol Hepatol (Paris) 21: 83–85
6. Burton MA, Gray BN, Jones C, Coletti A (1989) Intraoperative dosimetry of ^{90}Y in liver tissue. Int J Rad Appl Instrum [B] 16: 495–498
7. Houle S, Yip TK, Shepherd FA, Rotstein LE, Sniderman KW, Theis E, Cawthorn RH, Richmond-Cox K (1989) Hepatocellular carcinoma: pilot trial of treatment with Y-90 microspheres. Radiology 172: 857–860
8. Bretagne JF, Raoul JL, Bourguet P, Duvauferrier R, Deugnier Y, Faroux R, Ramee A, Herry JY, Gastard J (1988) Hepatic artery injection of I-131-labeled Lipiodol. II. Preliminary results of therapeutic use in patients with hepatocellular carcinoma and liver metastases. Radiology 168: 547–550
9. Raoul JI, Bretagne JF, Caucanas JP, Pariente EA, Boyer J, Paris JC et al. (1992) Internal radiation therapy for hepatocellular carcinoma. Results of a French multicenter phase II trial of transarterial injection of iodine 131-labeled Lipiodol. Cancer 69: 346–352
10. Mach JP, Bischof-Delaloye A, Curchod S, Studer A, Grob JP, Volant JC, Mosimann F, Givel JC, Douglas P, Leyvraz S et al. (1987) L'immunoscintigraphie par les anticorps monoclonaux radiomarqués. Evolution d'une méthode de diagnostic du cancer et espoir d'une nouvelle forme de thérapie. Schweiz Med Wochenschr 117: 1076–1086
11. Müller-Gartner HW, Montz R, Klapdor R, Hirschmann M, Rehpenning W, Langkowski J (1988) Radioimmunbehandlung solitärer Lebermetastasen mittels intratumoraler Instillation ^{131}J-markierter monoklonaler Antikörper—erste Ergebnisse einer klinischen Studie. Nuklearmedizin 27: 258–265
12. Barone RM, Calabro-Jones P, Thomas TN et al. (1981) Surgical adjuvant therapy in colon carcinoma: a human tumor spheroid model for evaluating radiation sensitizing agents. Cancer 47: 2349–2357
13. Moertel DG, Childs PS, Reitmeier PJ et al. (1969) Combined 5-fluorouracil and supervoltage radiation therapy of locally unresectable gastrointestinal cancer. Lancet 2: 865–867
14. Webber BM, Soderberg CH, Leone LA et al. (1978) A combined treatment approach to management of hepatic metastases. Cancer 42: 1087–1095
15. Wiley AL Jr, Wirtanen GW, Stephenson JA, Ramirez G, Demets D, Lee JW (1989) Combined hepatic artery 5-fluorouracil and irradiation of liver metastases. A randomized study. Cancer 64: 1783–1789
16. Raju PI, Maruama Y, De Simone P, MacDonald J (1987) Treatment of liver metastases with a combination of chemotherapy and hyperfractionated external radiation therapy. Am J Clin Oncol 10: 41–43
17. Gansl RC, Hippolito J, Cutait R et al. (1986) Treatment of liver metastatic colorectal carcinoma with sequential methotrexate (MTX), fluorouracil (5-FU), and external hepatic radiation. Proc Am Soc Clin Oncol 5: 94
18. Friedman MA, Cassidy MJ, Levine M et al. (1979) Combined modality therapy of hepatic metastases. Cancer 44: 906–913
19. Stillwagon GB, Order SE, Guse C, Klein JL, Leichner PK, Leibel SA, Fishman EK (1989) 194 hepatocellular cancers treated by radiation and chemotherapy combinations: toxicity and

response: a Radiation Therapy Oncology Group study. Int J Radiat Oncol Biol Phys 17: 1223–1229

20. Yoshikawa M, Ebara M, Ohto M, Miyoshi T (1990) A combination treatment of transcatheter arterial embolization (TAE) and irradiation for hepatocellular carcinoma (HCC) – evaluation for therapeutic efficacy in comparison with TAE or irradiation alone. Nippon Shokakibyo Gakkai Zasshi 87: 225–234

6 Ethanol Injection Therapy of Liver Tumors

Absolute ethanol is a powerful sclerosing agent that coagulates proteins, inducing immediate coagulation necrosis and partial or total vascular thrombosis. Necrosis is followed by formation of a granulation tissue and fibrosis. Ethanol is used in the treatment of kidney and liver cysts and for blockade of the celiac plexus, for example, in pancreatic cancer [1–3]. In embolotherapy, ethanol is used to treat inoperable kidney tumors and to sclerose varices in portal hypertension [4], superficial or deep angiomas, or AV malformations. Ethanol injected percutaneously into lesions is now used to treat liver tumors.

6.1 Patient Selection

Patients with tumors smaller than 3–5 cm, easily visible with sonography, can benefit from this technique. Larger tumors have also been treated to reduce the tumor burden. No more than two lesions should be treated. Patients with ascites or a tendency to marked bleeding are excluded. Platelet counts should be higher than 40 000, and prothrombin times greater than 35%. Neoplasms located under the surface can also be treated [5].

6.2 Technique

After local anesthesia, the lesions are punctured under real-time sonography guidance with a 19- to 21-G Chiba type needle. Depending on the size of the lesions, 2–8 ml absolute ethanol is injected through the needle into the tumor. Real-time sonography permits precise localization of the tip of the needle and monitoring of the injection of ethanol, which shows up as a hyperechoic zone (Fig. 6.1). Sometimes droplets of ethanol can be seen passing into the venous channels around the lesion, with no clinical evidence of sequelae [6]. The procedure is repeated two or three times a week until the total amount of the injected ethanol reaches the calculated volume. Depending on the radius (r, in centimeters) the volume (V, milliliters) of ethanol to be injected is calculated

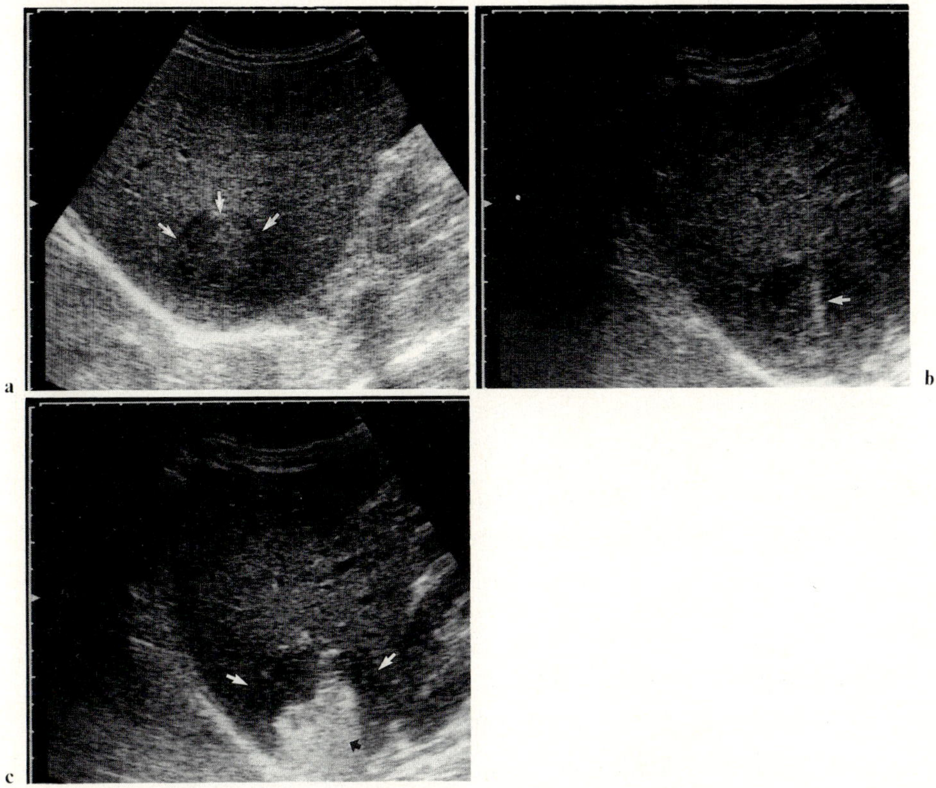

Fig. 6.1. a Hepatocellular carcinoma (*small white arrows*). **b** Alcoholization needle (*white arrow*) is within the tumor. **c** During ethanol injection. Note increasing echogenicity (*black arrow*) within tumor (*white arrows*)

using following formula: $V = 4/3\pi(r+0.5)^3$ ml. The total volume of ethanol can range from 4 to 95 ml. After the injections, hyperechoic lesions become hypoechoic or pseudocystic, and hypoechoic become isoechoic; lesions may disappear or calcify in the periphery.

Diffusion of ethanol has been studied experimentally [6] with methylene blue injected into focal tumors of surgical or necropsy material: (a) *in large tumors* the dye spreads along drainage channels, bypassing large areas of tumor tissue; (b) *in lesions of fibrous consistency* the dye remains in a circumscribed area, and several injections in different areas of the tumor must be performed to ensure sufficient diffusion; (c) *in lesions measuring less than 2 cm* the dye spreads through the whole tumor (this is also observed in some larger lesions).

Patients complain about local burning during and immediately after the injection. Pain is easily controlled with mild analgetics [6].

6.3 Results

In an analysis of 77 patients with hepatocellular carcinoma [7] the 1-, 2-, 3-, and 4-year survival rates were excellent: 89%, 74% 68%, and 60% respectively. Survival depended on liver function and on size of the largest lesion. Complications due to underlying cirrhosis (variceal bleeding and liver failure) were the most frequently encountered causes of death. Elevated α-fetoprotein levels decreased in 88% of patients; histopathological examinations performed in 14 cases showed the lesions to be totally necrotic in 10 (Fig. 6.2). In case of recurrence the treatment can be repeated. Metastases of cancers of different origin have also been successfully treated [6].

Complications are seldom encountered, but hemorrhage after tumor necrosis and liver abscess [8] have been described. Complications related to the fine needle puncture are extremely rare (see Chap. 3). No systemic side effects are encountered after ethanol injection.

Percutaneous ethanol injection of liver neoplasms is a valuable method for treatment of hepatocellular carcinomas. This technique probably also has a great potential (which has not yet be assessed in a randomized study) as a complement to chemoembolization. It may help treating the hypovascular

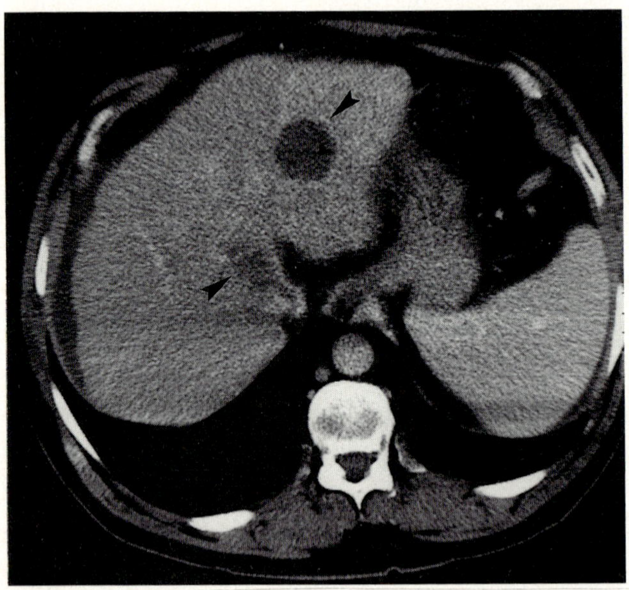

Fig. 6.2. Two hepatocellular carcinomas (*arrowheads*) in patient with alcoholic liver cirrhosis treated by ethanol injection alone in the lesion of the left lobe and by a combination of ethanol injection and chemoembolization in the lesion in the lobus caudatus. Note hypodensity and absence of enhancement indicative for necrosis. α-Fetoprotein reached normal levels at the end of treatment

parts of hepatic tumors or tumors out of reach of the catheter because of vascular anomalies. Compared with surgery [9], it seems the better treatment for hepatocellular carcinomas smaller than 3 cm and for lesions smaller than 5 cm in patients at high surgical risk [10]. The potential of alcoholization in treatment of metastases has still to be explored.

References

1. Bean WJ (1981) Renal cysts: treatment with alcohol. Radiology 138: 329–331
2. Haaga JR, Kori SH, Eastwood DW, Borkowski GP (1984) Improved technique for CT-guided celiac ganglia block. AJR Am J Roentgenol 142: 1201–1204
3. Solbiati L, Giangrande A, De Pra L, Belotti E, Cantù P, Ravetto C (1985) Percutaneous ethanol injection of parathyroid tumors under US guidance: treatment for secondary hyperparathyroidism. Radiology 155: 607–610
4. Yune HY, Klatte EC, Richmund BD, Olson EW, Becker GJ, Strickler SA (1985) Ethanol thrombotherapy of esophageal varices: further experience. AJR Am J Roentgenol 144: 1049–1053
5. Shiina S, Tagawa K, Unuma T, Fujino H, Uta Y, Hata Y, Niwa Y, Shiratori Y, Terano A, Sugimoto T (1990) Percutaneous ethanol injection therapy for neoplasms located on the surface of the liver AJR Am J Roentgenol 155(3) : 507–509
6. Livraghi T, Festi D, Monti F, Salmi A, Vettori C (1986) US-guided percutaneous alcohol injection of small hepatic and abdominal tumors. Radiology 161: 309–312
7. Shiina S, Tagawa K, Unuma T, Fujino H, Uta Y, Niwa Y, Hata Y, Komatsu Y, Shiratori Y, Terano A, Sugimoto T (1990) Percutaneous ethanol injection therapy of hepatocellular carcinoma: analysis of 77 patients. AJR Am J Roentgenol 155(6): 1221–1226
8. Isobe H, Fukai T, Iwamoto H, Satoh M, Tokumatsu M, Sakai H, Andoh B, Sakamoto S, Nawata H (1990) Liver abscess complicating intratumoral ethanol injection therapy for HCC. Am J Gastroenterol 85(12): 1646–1648
9. The Liver Cancer Study Group of Japan (1987) Primary liver cancer in Japan. Sixth report. Cancer 60: 1400–1411
10. Livraghi T, Vettori C (1990) Percutaneous ethanol injection therapy of hepatoma. Cardiovasc Intervent Radiol 13(3) : 146–152

7 Systemic Chemotherapy

7.1 Tumor Response to Chemotherapy

Systemic chemotherapy may be the appropriate treatment of liver metastases if the primary cancer is sensitive to chemotherapy. Metastases, however, are known to be sometimes less sensitive to chemotherapy than the primary tumor [1]. Depending on the nature of the neoplastic liver lesions, different rates of response to the treatment have been obtained.

Factors such as sex, age, performance status, extension of primary disease, time of diagnosis, and country of origin influence largely the natural history of disease and bias the outcome of therapeutic trials. Lead time bias (Fig. 7.1) due to improvement of diagnostic and imaging modalities can falsely show an increase in survival when treated groups of patients are compared to untreated patients of historical studies. Objective and comparable criteria must be used to determine response rates:

Stable disease
- Reduction of less than 50% in the product of the largest perpendicular diameters of the most clearly visible lesions

Partial response
- Reduction by at least 50% in the product of the largest perpendicular diameters of the most clearly visible lesions
- No increase in other lesions
- Absence of new areas of disease

Complete response
- Absence of any detectable tumor mass by any means, chemistry, radiographic studies

7.2 Hepatocellular Carcinomas

A variety of drugs have been used to treat hepatocellular carcinomas. In several controlled studies, no single chemotherapeutic agent showed superior activity. Response rates rarely reach 30% and often range about 10%. Survival rates achieved correspond to those obtained by placebos. Response rates obtained by various single agents are listed in Table 7.1.

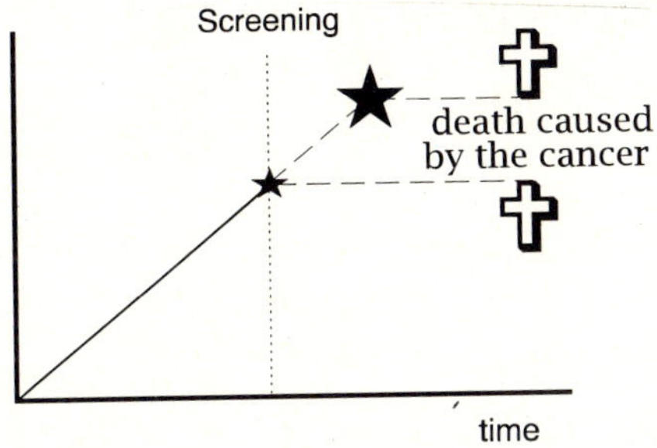

Fig. 7.1. Lead time bias

Table 7.1. Compilation of various clinical trials about response from hepatocellular carcinoma to single agent systemic chemotherapy (adapted and modified from [2])

Agent	*n*	No. of responses	Rate of responses %	Maximum mean survival
5-Fluorouracil iv	45	3	6.67	5 months
5-Fluorouracil po	66	6	9.09	2 months
Doxorubicin	484	77	15.91	4 months
Epirubicin	35	3	8.57	4 months
Neocarzinostatin	58	9	15.52	3 months
Etoposide	49	6	12.24	<3 months

Combination chemotherapy does not give results superior to those of single agents in clinical trials. Besides toxicity nothing is gained by adding chemotherapeutic drugs that by themselves do not show activity on the liver cancer to a cytostatic drug regimen. Results are disappointing, as shown in Table 7.2.

The relationship to anabolic steroids and oral contraceptive preparations, the male predominance among patients with cirrhosis, and the presence of estrogen receptors on tumor cells suggest that hepatocellular carcinoma may be a hormone-dependent tumor. Tamoxifen, an antiestrogen, was tested in several trials. A trial of doxorubicin and tamoxifen versus doxorubicin did not show any significant difference in survival or recurrence rate [7]. In a prospective controlled study comparing tamoxifen versus no treatment, a statistically significant increase in survival in tamoxifen-treated patients (22% versus 5% survival at 12 months) was reported. The α-fetoprotein level decreased, but tumor volume, lactate dehydrogenase, and alkaline phosphatase slowly increased. A slower, but continuous, progression of the disease was suggested [8]. Observers agree that

Table 7.2. Compilation of various clinical trials about response from hepatocellular carcinoma to combination of systemic chemotherapy (adapted and modified from [2])

Agent	*n*	Rate of responses %	Maximum mean survival
5-FU+MeCCNU [3]	55	13	<3 months
5-FU+STZ [3]	49	9	<3 months
5-FU+DOX [4]	38	13	3 months
5-FU+DOX+MeCCNU [3]	38	21	3 months
5-FU+DOX+MMC [5]	40	13	2 months
DOX+BLEO [6]	49	16	2 months

5-FU, Fluorouracil; MeCCNU, methyl-lomustine; STZ, streptozotocin; DOX, doxorubicin; MMC, mitomycin-C; BLEO, Bleomycin.

tamoxifen may be effective in the treatment of patients with hepatocellular carcinomas, but the exact role of tamoxifen, which is a well-tolerated drug, has still to be specified.

7.3 Liver Metastases

As mentioned in Sect. 7.1, systemic chemotherapy may be effective if the primary cancer is sensitive.

Treatment of liver metastases from colorectal carcinoma resulted in 22% of partial remissions in a trial of a dose-intensive regimen 5-fluorouracil (5-FU), consisting of bolus single-dose 5-FU therapy 400–500 mg, followed by 4-day infusion of 5-FU, 600–800 mg/m^2 per day, followed by a 17- to 24-day infusion of 200–250 mg/m^2 per day. Because of toxicity dose reduction was necessary in most patients [9]. Similar results with less toxicity may be achieved with combinations of leucovorin and 5-FU. In a prospective randomized trial, leucovorin significantly enhanced the therapeutic effect of 5-FU. Response rates of 30.3% were found versus 12.1% in the control group treated by 5-FU alone. Dose-limiting toxicity of the leucovorin plus 5-FU regimens was gastrointestinal, especially diarrhea [10].

Response rates greater than 30% are rarely attained and generally combined with considerable systemic toxicity (see Table 7.3). Metastases of other gastrointestinal malignancies such as pancreatic and gastric carcinomas also have a low response rate, ranging between 20% and 30%. Liver metastases from breast cancer are known to show high response rates, sometimes greater than 50%. A response rate of 55% in liver metastases after 120-h infusion of cisplatin and 5-FU was found in one trial [12], whereas equally high response rates were found using a regimen comprising cisplatin, doxorubicin, and cyclophosphamide [13].

Table 7.3. Compilation of various clinical trials about response from liver metastases from colorectal carcinoma to systemic chemotherapy (adapted and modified from [11])

Agent	No. of patients with liver metastases	Rate of liver response %
5-FU	165	22
5-FU + MeCCNU + VCR	189	21
5-FU + MeCCNU + VCR + STZ	89	34
5-FU + CF	73	30
5-FU + DDP + MMC + VCR	15	30
5-FU + DDP	99	19

5-FU, Fluorouracil; MeCCNU, methyl-lomustine; VCR, vincristine; STZ, streptozotocin; CF, leucovorin; MMC, mitomycin C; DDP, cisplatin.

References

1. Maehara Y, Sakaguchi Y, Emi Y, Kusumoto T, Kohnoe S, Mori M, Sugimachi K (1990) Primary and metastatic liver lesions of clinical colorectal cancer differ in chemosensitivity. Int J Colorectal Dis 5: 87–89
2. Wanebo HJ, Falkson G, Order S (1989) Cancer of the hepatobiliary tract. In: De Vita VT, Hellman S, Rosenberg SA (eds) Cancer. Principles and practice of oncology, 3rd edn. Lippincott, Philadelphia
3. Falkson G, Coetzer BJ, Terblanche APS (1984) Phase II trial of mitoxantrone in patients with primary liver cancer. Cancer Treat Rep Suppl 10, 68: 1311–1312
4. Baker LH, Saiki JH, Jones SE et al. (1977) Adriamycin and 5-fluorouracil in the treatment of advanced hepatoma. A Southwest Oncology Group study. Cancer Treat Rep 61: 1595–1597
5. Al-Hidrissi, Ibrahim E, Satir A et al. (1985) Primary hepatocellular cancer in the eastern province of Saudi Arabia: treatment with combination chemotherapy using 5-fluorouracil, Adriamycin and mitomycin-C. Hepatogastroenterology 32: 8–10
6. Ravery MJR, Omura GA, Bartolucci AA (1984) Phase II evaluation of epidoxorubicin plus bleomycin in hepatocellular carcinoma. A Southeastern Cancer Group trial. Cancer Treat Rep 68: 1517–1518
7. Melia WM, Johnson PJ, Williams R (1987) Controlled clinical trial of doxorubicin and tamoxifen versus doxorubicin alone in hepatocellular carcinoma. Cancer Treat Rep 71: 1213–1216
8. Farinati F, Salvagnini M, de Maria N, Fornasiero A, Chiaramonte M, Rossaro L, Naccarato R (1990) Unresectable hepatocellular carcinoma: a prospective controlled trial with tamoxifen. J Hepatol 11: 297–301
9. Poplin EA, Kraut M, Baker L, Brodfuehrer J, Vaitkevicius V (1991) A dose-intensive regimen of 5-fluorouracil for the treatment of metastatic colorectal carcinoma. Cancer 67: 367–371
10. Petrelli N, Douglass HO Jr, Herrera L, Russell D, Stablein DM, Bruckner HW, Mayer RJ, Schinella R, Green MD, Muggia FM et al. (1990) The modulation of fluorouracil with leucovorin in metastatic colorectal carcinoma: a prospective randomized phase III trial. Gastrointestinal Tumor Study Group. J Clin Oncol 7: 1419–1426 [Published erratum appears in J Clin Oncol (1990) 8: 185]

11. Kemeny N, Sugarbaker PH (1989) Treatment of metastatic cancer to liver. In: De Vita VT, Hellman S, Rosenberg SA (eds) Cancer. Principles and practice of oncology, 3rd Edn. Lippincott, Philadelphia
12. Fernandez Hidalgo O, Gonzalez F, Gil A, Campbell W, Barrajon E, Lacave AJ (1989) 120 hours simultaneous infusion of cisplatin and fluorouracil in metastatic breast cancer. Am J Clin Oncol 12: 397–401
13. Colozza M, Gori S, Mosconi AM, Belsanti V, Basurto C, Rossetti R, Di Costanzo F, Buzzi F, Bacchi M, Davis S et al. (1989) Chemotherapy with cis-platin, doxorubicin, and cyclophosphamide (CAP) in patients with metastatic breast cancer. Am J Clin Oncol 12: 137–141

8 Selective Perfusion of Chemotherapeutic Agents

8.1 General Considerations

8.1.1 Regional Chemotherapy: High Local Concentration of Drugs

As most chemotherapeutic drugs have a steep dose-response curve, the rationale for hepatic arterial infusion is to achieve a higher concentration of drugs in neoplastic lesions and to lower the systemic drug levels. Essays with labeled fluorodeoxyuridine (FUDR) show that drug concentration in neoplastic tissue after injection in the hepatic artery is nearly 15 times higher than after injection in the portal vein [1]. This study clearly demonstrates the advantage of administering regional chemotherapy through the hepatic artery, because tumorous areas in the liver obtain most of their blood supply from branches of the liver arteries whereas normal liver parenchyma is mainly supplied by the portal vein.

The advantage of regional chemotherapy can be quantified only with reference to systemic (generally intravenous) chemotherapy. The advantage of regional chemotherapy is seen the first time that the drug reaches the liver. When the drug leaves the liver, it reaches the systemic circulation and acts as systemically injected drugs. The advantage (A_{target}) in target concentration when injecting regionally versus systemically is determined by the ratio:

$$A_{target} = \frac{C_{target}(\text{regional})}{C_{target}(\text{systemic})}$$

The decrease ($D_{systemic}$) of systemic exposure to drugs injected regionally versus systemically is determined by:

$$D_{systemic} = \frac{C_{systemic}(\text{regional})}{C_{systemic}(\text{systemic})}$$

Selectivity for regional administration is defined by:

$$S = \frac{A_{target}}{D_{systemic}}$$

If an organ eliminates or metabolizes a drug delivered regionally, there is a first-pass effect. Where E is the fraction of drug eliminated by the target organ, the systemic concentration of drug that can be achieved is $1-E$. Thus:

$$D_{systemic}=\frac{C_{systemic}(\text{regional})}{C_{systemic}(\text{systemic})}=1-E$$

Two important factors influence the advantage (A_{target}) in target concentration of regionally injected drugs: local exchange rate and total body clearance of the drug. The local exchange rate (Q) describes fluid exchanges in a target organ. Typical values are listed in Table 8.1.The total body clearance (CL_{tb}) is specific to each drug. The advantage in target concentration of regionally injected drugs can thus be described as:

$$A_{target}=1+\frac{CL_{tb}}{Q}$$

Q, however, is a factor that can be reduced when drugs are administered intraarterially as reduction of flow by arterial ligature or embolization reduces Q and thus increases A_{target}. Increasing A_{target} is the one of the goals of combining regional chemotherapy and embolization (chemoembolization).

Combining the equations, selectivity for regional chemotherapy can be defined as:

$$S=1+\frac{CL_{tb}}{Q(1-E)}$$

When the target organ is also the organ that exclusively eliminates the drug:

$$S=\frac{1}{1-E}$$

Thus for regional chemotherapy to be effective selected drugs should have a high total-body clearance and be injected at sites with low regional exchange. Because of high regional exchange, drugs selected for intraarterial therapy should have a high clearance rate [2, 3]. 5-Fluorouracil (5-FU) and FUDR are drugs often used for regional chemotherapy in the liver. After the first pass 94–99% of FUDR is extracted, the extraction rate being higher after intraarterial injection than after portal injection. Advantage of regional delivery of various drugs is listed in Table 8.2. Advantages of intraarterial versus systemic administration of suitable chemotherapeutic agents in the liver are: (a) high

Table 8.1. Value of Q at various injection sites

Injection site	Q (ml/min)
Intrathecal	1
Intraperitoneal	10
Low flow intraarterial	100
High flow intraarterial	1000

Table 8.2. Drug advantage of selected chemotherapeutic drugs after regional infusion (adapted from [4])

Total-body clearance of drug (ml/min)	Drug	Regional drug delivery advantage
25 000	Fluorodeoxyuridine	101.0
4 000	5-Fluorouracil	17.0
3 000	Cytarabine	13.0
1 000	Carmustine	5.0
900	Doxorubicin	4.6
400	Cisplatin	2.6
200	Methotrexate	1.8

concentration of drugs reaching the tumorous tissue and (b) low systemic concentration of drugs especially for those with high first-pass extraction and high total-body clearance.

8.1.2 Anatomic Considerations: Vascular Remodeling

Regional chemotherapy can be performed in two different ways, the "radiological" or the "surgical." In the "radiological" way the catheter is positioned angiographically and withdrawn after each session of chemotherapy or chemoembolization. In the "surgical" way the catheter is implanted surgically. It is left in place for a long period, generally several months, and can be connected to an implantable pump or an injection port. Advantages and disadvantages of each technique are discussed below.

Before either type of catheter placement, surgical or radiological, a thorough analysis of the vascular anatomy of the liver must be performed as the anatomy of the celiac trunk and hepatic artery is subject to frequent variations. In a study of 200 cadavers, 41.5% had an aberrant artery, 31.5% having only one aberrant and 10% two and more [5]. Variations such as accessory hepatic arteries or hepatic arteries originating from the superior mesenteric arteries must be detected [6]. Because of numerous intrahepatic arterioarterial shunts, such aberrant arteries irrigating the liver may be ligated surgically or occluded angiographically by a Gianturco coil at their origin (Fig. 8.1). The arterial perfusion of the organ is not impaired as the distal part of the artery remains patent and is perfused through intrahepatic collaterals [7]. Vascular remodeling is most useful in obtaining a single artery irrigating the entire liver. When the left artery originates very proximally at the celiac trunk, it may be of interest to obstruct it, leaving only one main artery patent. Accessory arteries, such as right or left accessory hepatic arteries, can also be obliterated without problems. Reflux of chemotherapeutic agents (Fig. 8.2) in side branches is often a cause of complications. In our institution we try in each instance to obliterate the gastroduodenal artery at its origin with a 3- or 5-mm Gianturco coil. The perfusion of the

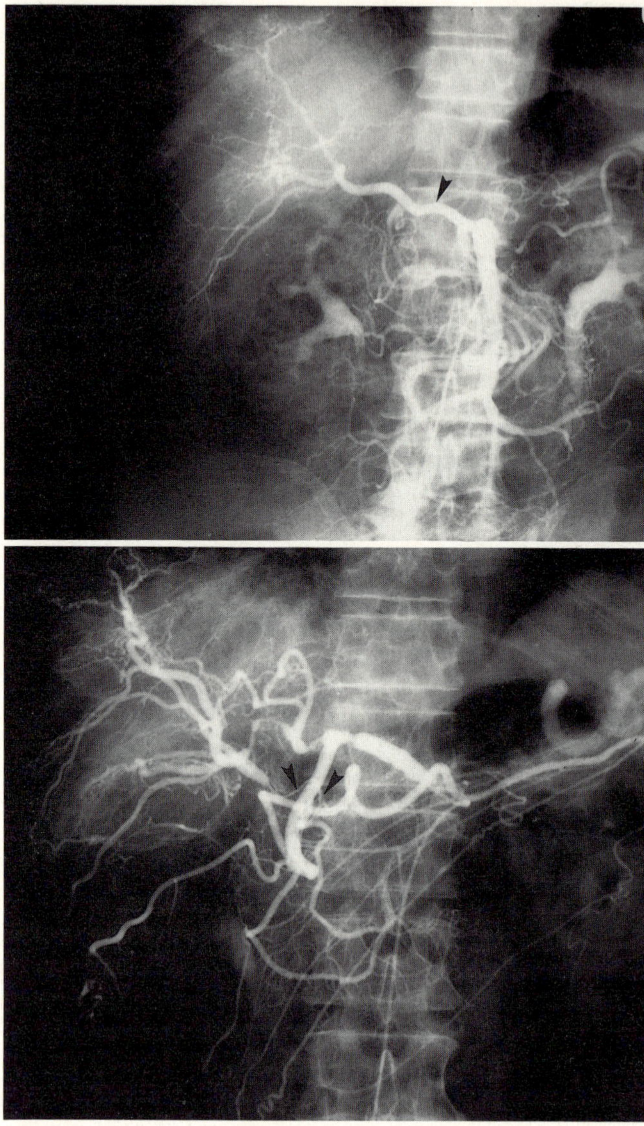

a

b

Fig. 8.1. **a** "Vascular remodeling." Right hepatic (*arrowhead*) comes from superior mesenteric artery. The rest of the liver is perfused normally by celiac trunk. **b** Catheter lies in common hepatic artery. The right hepatic artery was closed by a coil (*arrowheads*). Vascular "stenosis" is due to spasm. Branches distally from the coil are still patent and perfused by the common hepatic artery. "Vascular remodeling" transformed a liver with two main feeding arteries into a liver with a single feeding artery

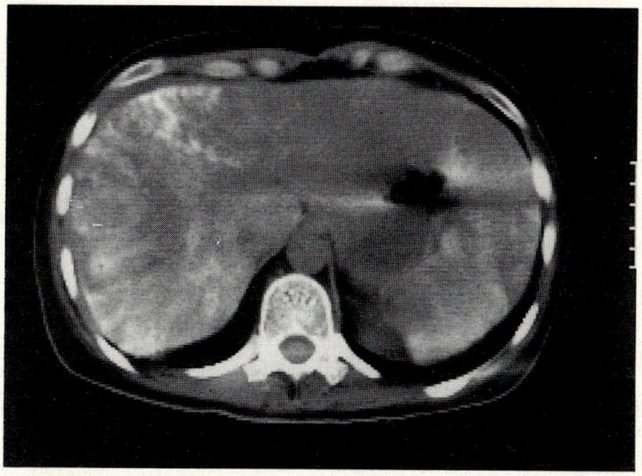

Fig. 8.2. Reflux of mixture of Lipiodol and chemotherapeutic agents in stomach and spleen (no consequences in this patient)

duodenal wall and pancreas head is ensured by anastomoses originating from the superior mesenteric artery (the pancreatico-duodenal arcades) and from the splenic artery.

8.1.3 Flow Pattern: Laminar Flow—Turbulent Flow

Typical flow in the hepatic artery is laminar. When droplets form at the tip of a catheter, they are driven by flow and sometimes follow the walls of the artery. Mixing of the chemotherapeutic agent with blood does not happen immediately; thus an important branch of the proper hepatic artery may be bypassed (for instance a lobar branch) and all of the agent may perfuse only one part of the liver. Movement of the patient or variation in blood pressure can alter the flow pattern, as was shown by a trial on effect of posture in drug distribution. Twelve patients had hepatic scintigraphy in supine and upright positions. Only 25% of scintigraphies were judged similar, 42% were slightly different, and 33% different [8]. Experimental work has shown that the time needed to mix a dye correctly in laminar flowing water is long, often too long to produce a homogeneous distribution through the liver. Rapid homogeneous mixing of the chemotherapeutic agent with the blood can be obtained by three means: (a) turbulent flow in the main arterial stream, (b) pulsed injection of the agent provoking small jets, or (c) high-volume injection of diluted chemotherapeutic agents at a high injection rate. Turbulent flow exists near arterial stenosis or plaques, but the hepatic artery itself is seldom as involved in arteriosclerotic processes as other arteries such as the renal, iliac, or carotid arteries. Stenoses can be artificially induced by the surgeon, but the flow pattern is still not under control because the exact location of the catheter tip in relation to the turbulent part of the flow, and the laminar flow cannot be determined. Pulsed flow as obtained by the Gianturco-Wallace chemotherapy pulser (COOK, Bloomingdale, USA) produces little jets of fluid at the tip of the catheter and thus a rapid mixing of the chemotherapeutic agent and blood. High injection volume at a high injection rate produces also an intimate mixing of the chemotherapeutic agent and blood.

8.1.4 Checking the Homogeneity of Liver Perfusion

To avoid complications and to obtain a homogeneous distribution of the chemotherapeutic agent throughout the liver, the tip of the catheter must be placed accurately according to the anatomy of the particular patient. Several techniques are used to check the homogeneity of the perfusion of the liver. Perfusion scintigraphy, using ^{99m}Tc macroaggregated albumin infused at 1 ml/min, is sensitive in detecting extrahepatic perfusion and is a good technique to determine the perfusion distribution in the whole liver. CT performed during slow injection of contrast medium through the intraarterial catheter is a more sensitive method than scintigraphy for the delineation of individual liver lesions, especially small ones, and for the evaluation of nonperfused areas of the liver. CT is less sensitive in detecting extrahepatic perfusion [9]. Digital subtraction angiography with a low injection rate of contrast (0.5 ml/s) is nearly as sensitive as scintigraphy with ^{99m}Tc macroaggregated albumin and superior to conventional angiography in predicting the extent of hepatic perfusion [10]. DSA and scintigraphy are the most sensitive modalities to define the presence or absence of extrahepatic perfusion.

None of the above imaging modalities entirely reflect reality. The rate of injection of contrast media or tracers is too high when compared to the typical chemotherapy infusion rate of 10 ml/h when using an implantable pump or an infusion port. The rate of injection during CT (1 ml/s) is 360 times, during DSA (0.5 ml/s) 180 times, and during perfusion scintigraphy (1 ml/min) 6 times higher than that of a chemotherapy infusion. As rapidity of mixture of chemotherapeutic agents and blood is partially flow rate dependent, the homogeneity of perfusion obtained using a pump under real-life conditions may not be the same as that documented by the various imaging modalities.

8.2 Regional Chemotherapy: The "Surgical Way"

Although many patients with hepatocellular carcinoma have benefited from regional chemotherapy with infusion in the hepatic artery, most of the work published concerns liver metastases of colorectal origin. This is not surprising because many primary cancers have metastases to the liver, but only colorectal cancer benefits from a very large database on natural history. Knowledge of the natural history of liver metastases of cancer of other origin such as breast, pancreas, and stomach is still insufficient to establish the value of different therapeutic modalities.

8.2.1 Intraarterial Regional Chemotherapy

Technique

Prior to catheter implantation, visceral angiography is performed to detect vascular variations. Most patients have a single artery to supply the liver, but a replaced right hepatic artery from the superior mesenteric artery is frequently found. By laparotomy under general anesthesia, the catheter is introduced through the gastroduodenal artery, the tip being placed in the hepatic artery. Access to the hepatic artery can also be gained through the splenic artery, the left gastric, or the gastroepiploic artery. The right gastric artery and branches to the duodenum and pancreas arising from the hepatic artery are ligated to reduce gastroduodenal side effects from chemotherapy. Patients with anatomical variants are treated by ligation of the non-dominant branches or by separate perfusion of the major branches. Complete perfusion of the whole liver is confirmed by intraoperative injection of fluorescein under ultra-violet light or by using macroaggregated ^{99m}Tc-labeled albumin and a gamma camera. Some teams systematically perform cholecystectomy to avoid chemical cholecystitis, while others do so only selectively. The catheters are connected either to an infusion port or to an implantable pump. Multiple cycles of FUDR or 5-FU are injected, sometimes combined with starch microspheres or with $15\,mg/m^2$ mitomycin C. Injection protocols vary from infusion over 1 week every two weeks to infusion every 2 weeks followed by 2 weeks of heparinized saline. FUDR is typically injected at daily doses of 0.2–0.3 mg/kg. Contraindications to intraarterial chemotherapy are extrahepatic disease, jaundice, leukopenia, thrombocytopenia, and underlying nonmalignant liver disease. A preoperative evaluation including CT scans of the abdomen and chest is needed to identify extrahepatic disease and to prevent unnecessary laparotomy [11].

Results

Results of intraarterial chemotherapy with surgically implanted catheters connected to pumps or infusion ports have been disappointing [12, 13]. Response rates depend on the criteria used, varying from 88% when the only criterion is a decrease of in carcinoembryonic antigen to 29% based on CT criteria. Partial response and stabilization rate is about 50% when the classical criteria described in Chap. 7 are used.

No proven increase in long-term survival has yet been found. Responders have a mean survival time of about 14–18 months, about twice that of nonresponders. Complete responders, if any, are very rare. Intraarterial chemotherapy produces a higher response rate than intravenous chemotherapy and may be effective even after failure of intravenous chemotherapy. One unsolved problem remains extrahepatic recurrence such as lung metastases, local adenopathy, and peritoneal carcinosis. Regional chemotherapy influences the natural history of liver metastases but does not significantly prolong survival as other patterns of manifestation appear. Most of the chemotherapeutic drugs injected in the artery are extracted and eliminated to a high degree by the liver itself. Recirculating drugs do not reach a concentration high enough efficiently to treat extrahepatic disease. Because of the fairly high degree of response, intraarterial chemotherapy is probably a good way to control the hepatic manifestation of cancer; the way to control extrahepatic disease has not yet been found.

Modern implantable pumps are reliable instruments with a low failure rate, and they have brought an increase in life quality compared to external perfusions through injection ports. However, the technique is hampered by a high rate of complications, related to the catheter, the pump, and the chemotherapy (see below). The absence of survival benefit and the high rate of complications has induced several groups to abandon this technique [14].

8.2.2 Portal Versus Intraarterial Chemotherapy

Arteriography and histological studies show that blood supply to liver tumors comes predominantly from the arterial system and a small but definite portion from the portal venous system. Infusion of chemotherapeutic agents in the portal vein would theoretically have some advantages, such as anatomical uniformity, easy peroperative cannulation, and low toxicity; however, tumor drug uptake after portal infusion is clearly inferior to that after arterial infusion [1].

In a randomized trial allowing crossover of the arms and designed to find the best infusion site for maximal tumor response, tumor response after intraarterial infusion was clearly superior compared with portal infusion [15].

As portal infusion has not been shown to be superior to systemic therapy, it no longer has any use for therapy of existing metastases, intraarterial perfusion being preferred to portal perfusion in clinical practice. The only instance in which portal infusion is still employed is in the perioperative period as adjuvant chemotherapy (see below).

8.2.3 Adjuvant Intraportal Chemotherapy for Colorectal Hepatic Metastases

Discovery of tumor cells in the mesenteric venous blood of 32% of patients during surgery for colorectal carcinoma [16] led to the now challenged [17] concept of "no-touch isolation technique" for tumor resection and later to the idea of adjuvant intraportal chemotherapy.

In an early randomized study, Taylor et al. [18] showed benefits of intraportal infusion of 7 g 5-FU during the first 7 postoperative days. After an observation of 28 months, 23 patients died in the control group but only 7 in the infusion group. Several controlled studies have been conducted since. In a study of 224 patients with resected Duke stage B2 or C colorectal cancer, randomized either to an untreated control group or to a group receiving 7 days of 5-FU therapy (500 mg/m^2 per day) by portal vein infusion, no benefit of the treatment was found in terms of interval to progression and survival curves [19]. In a Swiss study including 469 patients, a control group was compared with patients receiving 500 mg/m^2 5-FU per day with heparin for 7 days and 10 mg mitomycin C on day 1. The 5-year survival was 70% versus 57% and the absence of recurrence of 62% versus 53% in favor of the treated group [20]. A Dutch prospective study [21] involved 304 patients with colorectal cancer randomized to three groups, 1 g 5-FU plus heparin per day for 7 days versus 240×10^3 U urokinase per day for 7 days versus a control group. The group treated by intraportal chemotherapy had significantly fewer patients with liver metastases than the control group (7% versus 23%). There was, however, no significant improvement in the mortality associated with portal 5-FU therapy.

Other studies show no benefit of adjuvant intraportal chemotherapy, or small advantages in the absence of recurrence. The therapy is considered safe and without substantial side effects. Increase in surgical complications or mortality has not been demonstrated. Considering available information, intraportal infusion cannot be recommended in clinical practice [22]: the definite proof of its utility and benefits in long-term survival is still lacking. All patients receiving adjuvant chemotherapy should be included in study protocols. The NIH Consensus Conference (16–18 April 1990) recommended [23] the use of Intergroup protocol with 5-FU and levamisole [24] for patients in stage III who are not included in clinical studies.

8.2.4 Adjuvant Intraperitoneal Chemotherapy for Colorectal Hepatic Metastases

Besides liver metastases, local recurrence and peritoneal seeding following surgery are major problems in the treatment of colorectal cancer. Local recurrence and peritoneal seeding are found mostly in autopsy series and at reoperation, as radiological techniques often fail to demonstrate them.

5-FU, doxorubicin, or cisplatin, diluted in large volumes of dyalisate, are infused through a Tenkoff catheter implanted after completion of surgery to remove the primary intestinal cancer. The drugs, which have only a limited penetration in peritoneal tumor deposits, reach plasmatic levels corresponding to 30% of bolus injections and up to 20 times those of continuous infusions over 24 h. Tenkoff catheters induce a fibrotic reaction, which combined with the adhesive effect of surgery prevent uniform intraabdominal drug delivery. Also, some of the agents themselves induce fibrosis [25].

In a prospective, randomized trial comparing intravenous versus intraperitoneal 5-FU, the natural history of surgically treated colorectal cancer was changed by the significant reduction in the incidence of peritoneal carcinomatosis. There was no difference, however, in survival or time before relapse. Intraperitoneal infusion significantly reduced hepatic and hematological toxicity, and the tolerable dose of drugs was increased without an increase in side effects [26].

After resection of hepatic colorectal metastases, intraperitoneal adjuvant chemotherapy did not influence patient survival [27], although high intraportal levels of 5-FU (but not of mitomycin C) were measured [28]. The lack of effect on hepatic metastases should not be astonishing as direct portal perfusion did not show a significant effect on survival of patients with liver metastases. Intraperitoneal infusion should thus be limited to clinical trials for patients at high risk for progression of peritoneal carcinomatosis

8.3 Regional Chemotherapy: The "Radiological" Way

Until now most work published on regional chemotherapy using the "radiological" way has centered on treatment of hepatocellular carcinoma. Experience in treating liver metastases with these techniques is not as great as that with the "surgical" way.

In the first session of regional chemotherapy using the radiological approach, a complete angiographic workup is performed, including selective angiography of the celiac trunk, splenic artery, common hepatic artery, and superior mesenteric artery. Portal circulation is analyzed. In our institution, when possible, we try to catheterize the gastroduodenal artery with a 5-F catheter and to place a 3- or 5-mm Gianturco coil at its origin to avoid later inadvertent perfusion or embolization to the pancreas or the duodenum. At the beginning of following sessions we routinely perform angiography of the celiac trunk to check the integrity of the arterial and portal tree.

Usually the right femoral artery is punctured using the Seldinger technique. After positioning the 6-F introducer, a 5-F catheter is advanced and placed in the proper hepatic artery. We routinely use a single-curve polyethylene catheter (COOK, Bloomingdale, USA) or a 5-F catheter designed at our institution (Hoogewoud Superselective catheter, COOK, Denmark) with a long floppy tip. We systematically use steerable guide wires with a hydrophylic coating for selective or superselective angiography. Usually the combination of a catheter with a floppy tip and a steerable guide wire with hydrophylic coating permits superselective catheterization of segmental or subsegmental branches of the hepatic arteries. When the celiac trunk and its branches are very tortuous, a 2.2-F coaxial Tracker microcatheter system (Target Therapeutics, San Jose, CA, USA) allows one to overcome anatomical difficulties.

Table 8.3. Typical duration of a chemoembolization session and of fluoroscopy at our institution

Procedure	Duration	Fluoroscopy time
Placement of perfusion catheter	40 min	7 min
Chemoembolization	70 min	12 min
First session with embolization of the gastroduodenal artery	90 min	16 min

After chemoembolization, the catheter is withdrawn. When perfusion is preferred, the catheter is positioned so as to ensure perfusion of the whole liver. The catheter is attached to the skin by a single stitch and left in place for 24 h.

DSA is most useful to speed up the whole procedure. The angiographic equipment that we use (Philips DVI S, Philips, Best, Netherlands) has a remote control pad that gives the angiographer nearly full control of the machine. The average duration of typical sessions and of fluoroscopy at our institution is shown in Table 8.3.

8.3.1 Intraarterial Perfusion

The catheter in the femoral artery is connected to an electronic infusor with which 1000 ml saline per day containing 5000 U/l heparin is infused continuously to keep the catheter patent. At our institution we dilute the chemotherapy drug in 250 ml saline and inject it over 30 min (8.33 ml/min). The Gianturco-Wallace chemotherapy infusor is systematically used to ensure complete mixing of drugs with blood intraarterially. Smaller amounts of drugs are injected by hand, with little pushes on the piston of the syringe, to ensure turbulent flow at the tip of the catheter. An intravenous line is also placed for the injection of antiemetics or systemic chemotherapy when needed. The patient remains in bed until the whole protocol, usually lasting 24 h, is completed and the hepatic catheter withdrawn. For the whole treatment the patient remains 2–3 days in hospital.

Results of intraarterial perfusion using the "radiological" way are similar to those using the "surgical" way. The technique-related complication rate is, however, lower; there are fewer catheter-related complications, fewer thromboses of the hepatic artery, and no pump-related complications. Further, there is no need for laparotomy when metastases are discovered after surgery of the primary tumor has been performed.

Generally the classical chemotherapeutic agents such 5-FU, mitomycin, cisplatin, and doxorubicin are used for intraarterial perfusion. Other intraarterially injected agents such recombinant human tumor necrosis factor, with a low objective response rate of 14%, have been used on patients with chemotherapy-resistant disease [29].

8.3.2 Chemotherapeutic Drugs and Lipiodol

After injection of a drug in the hepatic artery, healthy liver parenchyma takes up a part and metabolizes it, the cancer takes up a part, and the rest recirculates. The use of a carrier has the effect of retaining the drug in the liver, to slowly release it and increase its concentration locally. Lipiodol (Laboratoires Guerbet, Aulnay-sous-Bois, France), a contrast medium based on iodized poppy seed oil and used for lymphography, is the carrier most frequently used. The drugs can either be injected as a suspension, prepared by dispersing the drug directly into Lipiodol, or as an emulsion, obtained by emulsifying an aqueous solution of the drug into the lipid contrast medium. Drug release seems to be more prolonged in suspensions than in emulsions. Tumors often accumulate the oily contrast medium (Fig. 8.3) which leaks out of the vascular spaces and attaches to the cancerous cell membrane as a nonglobular lipid and enters the cancerous cell as a globular lipid [30]. Contrast medium in excess in normal parenchyma is eliminated by macrophages and hepatic lymphatic drainage. Accumulation of Lipiodol in the tumor cell (an effect used to detect small nodules of hepatocellular carcinomas in Lipiodol CT; see Chap. 3) has the effect of increasing the concentration of the drugs intracellularly. Significant amounts of doxorubicin

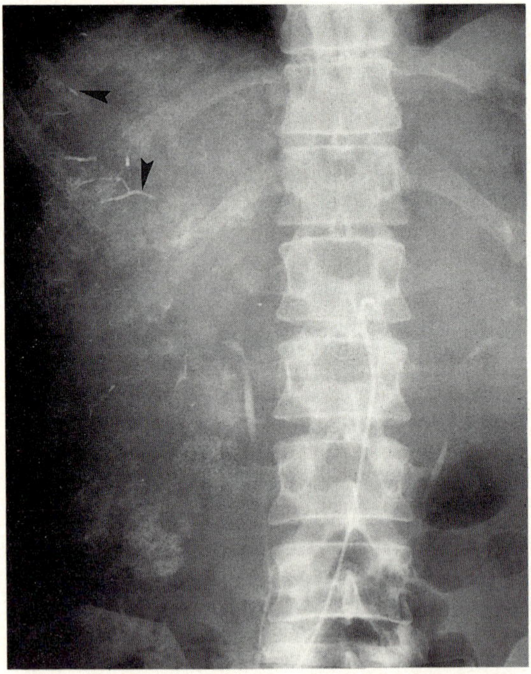

Fig. 8.3. Accumulation of Lipiodol in hepatic metastastases. Branching opacities (*arrowheads*) are vessels filled with a mixture of Ivalon, Lipiodol, and chemotherapeutic agents

have been found in liver specimens resected from patients 1 and 2 months after injection of doxorubicin plus Lipiodol [31]. As Lipiodol is a contrast medium, it acts like a tracer. CT scans performed after injection show the homogeneity of the drug distribution throughout the liver. The parts receiving insufficient doses of drugs are the focus of particular attention during the next session of chemoembolization.

8.3.3 Embolization

Embolization is a technique used to occlude temporarily or permanently parts or the totality of a vascular tree so as to check a hemorrhage, induce an ischemic necrosis, or stop the development of a vascular malformation. The choice of material used for embolization depends on the goal to be achieved. Liquid agents such as ethanol or histacryl reach the capillary level and induce a definite occlusion of the vascular tree. Particulate material reaches small arteries the size of which depends on the size of the particles. Pieces of resorbable material such as Gelfoam induce a temporary occlusion, the arteries generally being recanalized after a few weeks. Table 8.4 lists materials most frequently used for embolization.

In embolization of liver neoplasms, liquid agents are not used, particulate material such as Ivalon, Gelfoam powder or particles being preferred. Liquid agents can pass neoplastic arteriovenous shunts and have systemic effects. Particulate material is retained by the tumor arterioles (Fig. 8.4). Caution must be given in the presence of large shunts as smaller particles can flow through and reach the lungs.

The effects of embolization of liver tumors are manifold. Embolization in itself, when complete, is effective in the treatment of neoplastic lesions, provided the size of the material used for embolization is small enough to reach the center

Table 8.4. Type and properties of materials used for embolization

Material	Temporary occlusion	Permanent occlusion	Proximal occlusion	Distal occlusion
Liquids				
Ethanol	No	Yes	Yes	Yes
Sclerosing agents	No	Yes	Yes	Yes
Histacryl	No	Yes	Yes	Yes
Particulate				
Gelfoam powder	Sometimes	Yes	Yes	Yes
Gelfoam particles	Yes	Sometimes	Yes	No
Ivalon	No	Yes	Yes	Depends on particle size
Coils	No	Yes	Yes	No
Balloons	No	Yes	Yes	No

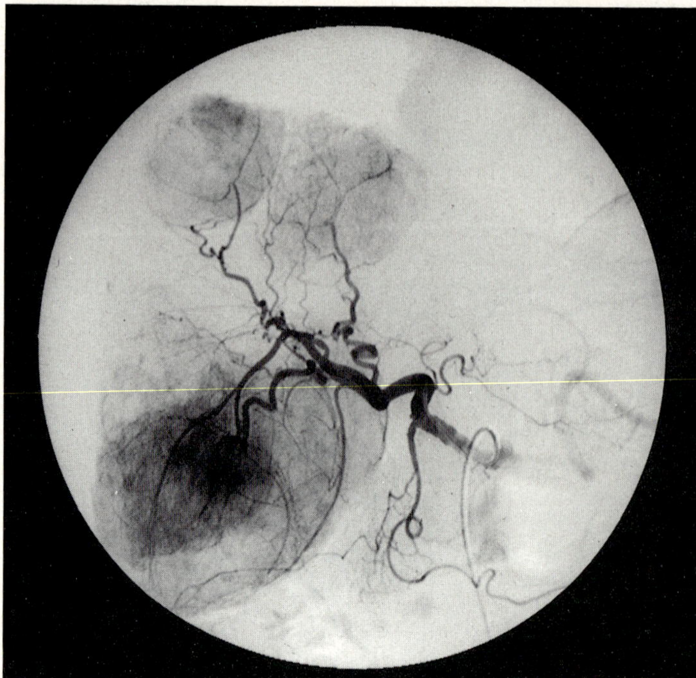

a

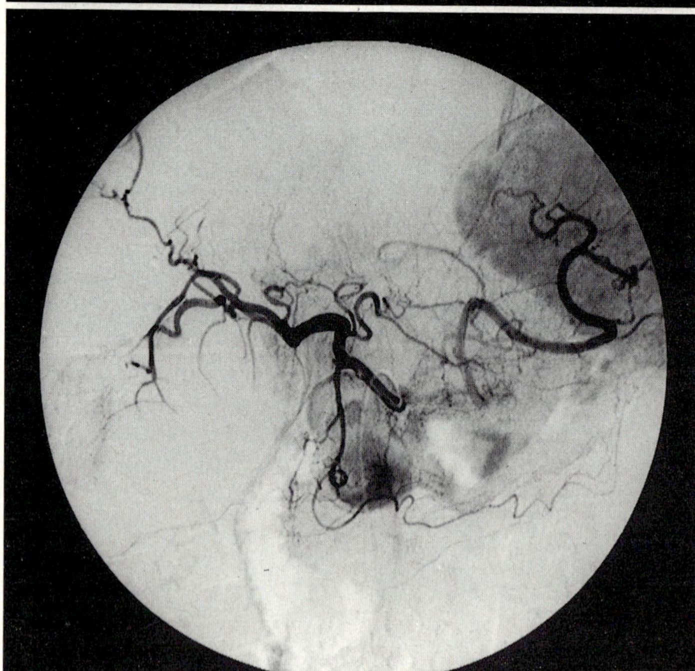

b

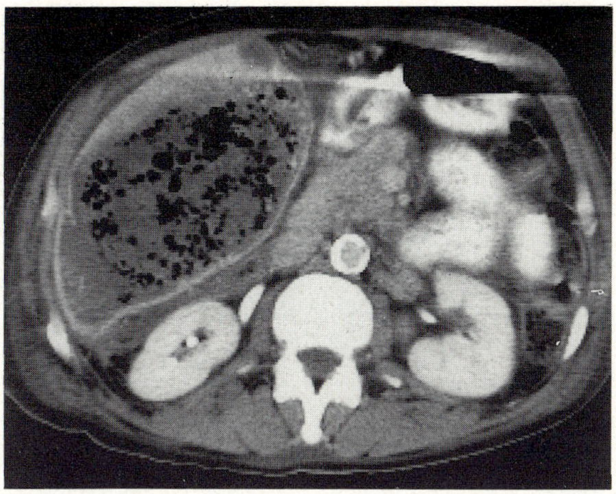

Fig. 8.5. Extensive necrosis of large hepatocellular carcinoma of right liver lobe. Note extensive gas formation in necrotic tumor. This picture may be misinterpreted as abcess. Multiples biopsies showed only presence of necrotic tumor

of the lesion. If this condition is fulfilled, ischemic necrosis is induced. Necrosis can easily be followed-up on CT scans; lesions become hypodense, do not enhance after contrast injection, and often contain gas bubbles after a few days (Fig. 8.5). Best results are obtained with richly vascularized tumors such as neuroendocrine tumors. Because of arterial flow reduction, embolization slows release of chemotherapeutic drugs mixed with Lipiodol and increases the advantage of regional chemotherapy.

Embolization is also very effective in stopping intraperitoneal hemorrhage in cases of spontaneous rupture of hepatocellular carcinomas [32].

8.3.4 Chemoembolization

Chemoembolization is a combination of intraarterial chemotherapy and embolization. With this technique one tries to combine the cytotoxic effect of the chemotherapeutic drugs with the effects of embolization: necrosis through ischemia, increase in cytotoxicity through increased local concentration, and slow release of drugs because of diminished washout (Fig. 8.6). The technique generally in use consists of injecting a mixture of 5–10 ml Lipiodol and of a chemotherapeutic drug first and embolizing with Gelfoam particles afterwards (sandwich therapy) until the arterial flow is markedly reduced or stops.

Fig. 8.4. **a** Neuroendocrine liver metastases. **b** After chemoembolization. Note devascularization of metastases, but most main liver arteries are still patent. Ivalon was used as embolic agent

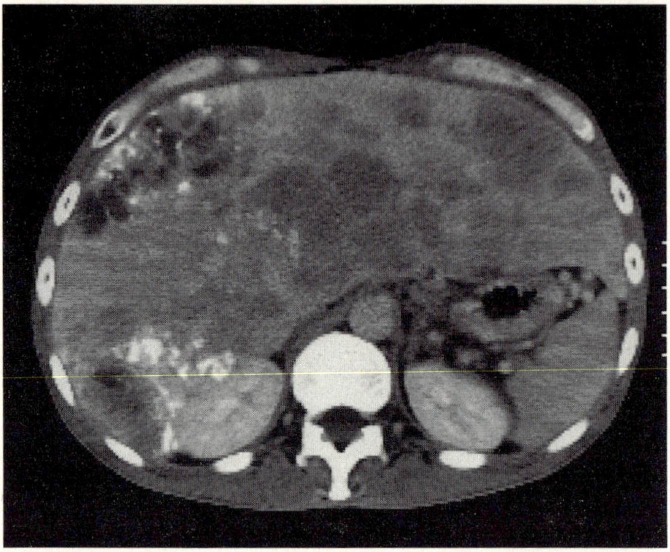

Fig. 8.6. Metastastic liver treated by chemoembolization only of the right liver; vascular anomalies hindered catheterization of left liver. There is extensive necrosis of nodules of right liver with accumulation of hyperdense Lipiodol. Recirculating chemotherapeutic agents had no effect on left liver nodules

Recanalization of the occluded artery occurs after a short time, generally a few weeks. There are many variations of this technique. We prefer to use Ivalon and when possible to embolize more selectively. The protocols employed in our institution are listed in Table 8.5.

Microspheres loaded with chemotherapy drugs or microencapsulated drugs [33] have also been injected. Another variation of this technique consists of injecting radioactive ^{90}Y [34] (discussed in Chap. 5).

Patient Selection, Indications, Contraindications

Patients with nonresectable liver lesions can be selected for intraarterial perfusion or chemoembolization. The embolization part of the treatment must be confined to patients with a patent portal system and a documented hepatopetal flow. Patients with partially occluded portal veins or with hepatofugal flow depend on arterial flow and are at risk of liver failure due to liver ischemia or infarction. Exceptionally, depending on the configuration of the tumor and the arterial supply of the tumor as well as on the skill of the angiographer, the tumor may be treated by chemoembolization when the catheter is placed superselectively. Liver failure, absence of hepatopetal portal flow, and thrombosis of the portal vein are absolute contraindications of chemoembolization. Perfusion alone without embolization may be discussed from case to case. Because of the

Table 8.5. Chemoembolization protocols

	Liver metastases colorectal	Liver metastases of other origin	Hepatocellular carcinoma
Cytostatics		Cytostatics mixed with 5–10 ml Lipiodol adapted to the type of tumor and injected at their normal (systemic) doses	
		or	
	1000–1500 mg 5-FU mixed with 5 ml Lipiodol *and* 15–30 mg mitomycin C mixed with 5 ml Lipiodol *and/or* 60 mg cisplatin	30 mg mitomycin C mixed with 5 ml Lipiodol *and* 100 mg cisplatin mixed with 5 ml Lipiodol	40–60 mg doxorubicin mixed with 5–10 ml Lipiodol
Embolization material	250–1000 mg Ivalon 250–500 μm until slowing down of flow *and/or* Gelfoam particles	250–1000 mg Ivalon 250–500 μm until slowing down of flow *and/or* Gelfoam particles	250–1000 mg Ivalon 250–500 μm until slowing down of flow *and/or* Gelfoam particles

Protocols with doses for one session of chemoembolization of the liver used in Cantonal Hospital, Fribourg. The sessions may be repeated. If reduced flow is still observed during the subsequent session(s), less embolization material is injected. The given values correspond to a normalized individual of 1.73 m^2 and 75 kg. Doses are adapted in each case.

risk of infection, biliary obstruction is a relative contraindication to chemoembolization, except for cases in which the treatment can relieve the obstacle [35].

In selected cases, chemoembolization in patients with inoperable hepatocellular carcinoma leads to resectability of the lesion. Preoperative chemoembolization of hepatocellular carcinomas can influence favorably the recurrence rate and the survival rate [36, 37]. No viable tumor was found in 40% of patients with hepatocellular carcinomas treated preoperatively with cisplatin, Lipiodol, and Gelfoam sponge, marked necrosis of the tumor being found in the remainder [38]. In patients with resectable hepatocellular carcinomas, chemoembolization is considered useful in preventing tumor growth, thickening the capsule, and thus making surgery safer–also reducing the chances of recurrence [39]. However, the favorable influence of preoperative chemoembolization of hepatocellular carcinomas is challenged by some authors as the tumors are sometimes not found intraoperatively, and the operation is sometimes needlessly complicated [40]. Gangrenous changes of the gallbladder and adhesions of the hepatoduodenal ligament have been described [41].

Results

Because of the different nature of these tumors, treatment results in hepatocellular carcinomas and in metastases of endocrine tumors and of other types are discussed separately. The classical response criteria are listed in Table 7.1.

These internationally accepted criteria are not complete. They do not take into account biopsy-confirmed total necrosis of liver tumors transformed into cystoid liquid structures of the same size as the original tumor (Fig. 8.7). This type of response is frequently found with chemoembolization.

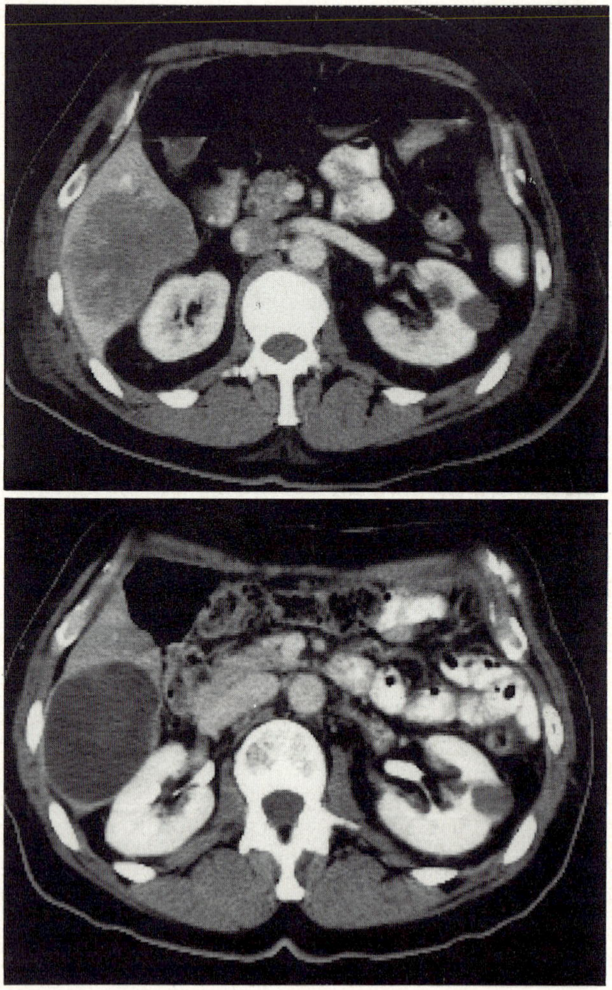

Fig. 8.7. Cytic necrosis of metastasis. Metastasis of colorectal cancer before treatment and 9 months later. Note cystic degeneration of tumor. Multiple biopsies showed absence of viable tumor

Results of studies about treatment of liver tumors must be interpreted very carefully. Differences in survival among untreated patients depend on various factors such as subtype of tumors, extension, rate of replacement of the liver, and liver function. Survival rates or response rates are often biased by patient selection.

Hepatocellular Carcinomas

Japanese authors have the greatest experience in chemoembolization of hepatocellular carcinomas. Several thousand patients have already been treated. Because of the lack of controlled stratified studies, benefits in survival are difficult to establish. Although there is evidence of a local effect of chemoembolization or intraarterial chemotherapy, the effect of these techniques on long-term survival is still not proven. It is now well known that there are important variations in the survival of untreated patients with hepatocellular carcinomas. Encephalopathy, male sex, older age, jaundice, alcohol consumption, elevated α-fetoprotein and bilirubin levels negatively influence survival [42–44]. Differences can often be explained by patient selection, hepatocellular carcinoma subtype, or other prognostic factors. Controlled, stratified studies including all patients, as well as postoperative and early deaths, must still be carried out.

It seems that chemoembolization benefits only a selected group of patients with unresectable cancer, limited disease, and cirrhosis. If the tumor invades portal branches, is hypovascular, or occupies more than 20% of the liver parenchyma, survival is not different from that in patients treated only conservatively [45]. In a randomized study, 42 patients with unresectable hepatocellular carcinoma and no contraindication for chemoembolization were divided in two groups: one treated by repeated chemoembolization with Gelfoam powder and doxorubicin and the other treated symptomatically. The groups were homogeneous in terms of liver function, age, and stage of cirrhosis. Although no significant difference in survival was noted, there were some complete or partial responses [46].

In a series about 100 patients with small hepatocellular carcinomas treated with either surgery, arterial embolization, or intraarterial chemotherapy, the median survival was, without considering the type of treatment, 37.1 months for Child A patients, 16.2 months for Child B patients, and 1.6 months for Child C patients (Child's classification for estimation of hepatic reserve is presented in Table 4.1). Analyzing the effects of the major therapeutic modalities on survival with regard to Child's grading, surgery was recommended in Child A patients, arterial embolization in Child B patients, and no treatment in Child C patients [47]. The result of this study confirms that patients with small hepatocellular carcinomas and intact liver function have a better chance of survival, and that surgical resection is probably the best treatment for this group. Comparing surgery with percutaneous ethanol injection in this homogeneous group of patients would be of interest, as the efficiency of ethanol on small hepatocellular carcinomas is proven, and no functional liver parenchyma is lost as is the case with resection surgery.

Five-year survival is about 10%. Although the tumor control rate is higher, deaths are often due to complications of the underlying cirrhosis such as variceal bleeding or liver failure or to extrahepatic recurrence.

Embolization and chemoembolization are efficient in treating symptoms caused by hepatocellular carcinomas. Pain, fever, and paraneoplastic hypercalcemia can be controlled in about 60%–70% of patients [48, 49]. Hemorrhage after spontaneous rupture of hepatocellular carcinomas can be controlled in most patients, provided portal blood flow is maintained [50, 51].

With chemoembolization it is possible to induce marked necrosis in hepatocellular carcinomas. Surgery performed after chemoembolization shows subtotal necrosis or even total disappearance of the tumor. Unfortunately, residual tumor related to small satellite lesions, extracapsular extension, or portal vein involvement is often found [52]. Although chemoembolization is effective, presence of viable residual tumor is an argument for surgical resection. Massive nodular disease considered to be non-resectable can be converted to a resectable state by chemoembolization [53].

The effect of chemoembolization can be monitored by the decrease of the α-fetoprotein level, which reaches normal values in about 43% and decreases more than 50% in about 27% of cases [54].

Treatment of lesions located in the caudate lobe is difficult because the origins of the arterial branches are rarely recognized on angiograms. Results of chemoembolization of lesions located in the caudate lobe are poor [55].

Although the main hepatic tumor can be controlled by chemoembolization, cancer may progress due to local lymphatic metastases and distant metastases. Because of hepatic retention and excretion, the doses and concentration of the recirculating part of chemotherapeutic agents is insufficient to treat these metastases. Small intrahepatic metastases and daughter nodules do not have capsules and are resistant to embolization [56].

Survival should not be the only argument for or against chemoembolization. Palliation, control of symptoms such as pain or fever, and quality of life are elements to be discussed among the indications for chemoembolization. Using a questionnaire, a Japanese group established that chemoembolization and intraarterial perfusion, compared to symptomatic treatment, favorably influences life quality. These techniques also help in maintaining patients at home for a longer period [57].

Summary

In the treatment of hepatocellular carcinomas chemoembolization is an effective modality for palliation and life quality. Survival may be favorably influenced in selected patients, but confirmation of survival prolongation is still lacking.

Except for the group of small hepatocellular carcinomas, which can be treated by percutaneous injection of ethanol, chemoembolization appears to be the best nonsurgical treatment of hepatocellular carcinomas. It should be reserved for a selected group of patients, namely symptomatic patients or patients with a patent portal vein, hepatopetal flow, and graded Child A or B grading. Although there is no real proof of an effect on survival, there are long-term survivors among the patients treated by chemoembolization; they are virtually nonexistent in the group of untreated patients.

Treatment of Metastases of Neuroendocrine Tumors

Because of the rarity of the condition, published series on embolization, chemoembolization, or intraarterial chemotherapy are small. All confirm, however, that hormonal activity of metastases of neuroendocrine tumors can be effectively controlled by these techniques. In a series of ten patients with islet cell or carcinoid tumors treated by embolization, all patients improved almost immediately. There was a measurable decrease in hormonal levels or tumor size [58]. In a small series of six patients with malignant carcinoid tumors, embolization produced noticeable relief of symptoms especially facial flushing and diarrhea. Embolization was repeated in three of six patients. Embolization of liver metastases from neuroendocrine tumors is considered a safe and repeatable method to palliate symptoms of hormonal secretion [59, 60].

Treatment of Metastases of Other Tumors

Many studies have been published on regional chemotherapy of liver metastases, especially of colorectal origin and generally using the surgical approach, but few studies exist about chemoembolization. Again, Japanese authors have the greatest experience in this field. Results of chemoembolization (Fig. 8.8) seem to be slightly better than those of regional chemotherapy with implanted catheters. Although not statistically significant, survival compared to infusion chemotherapy seems to be favorably influenced [61]. The overall survival rate remains disappointing. In a series about 68 patients the 6-month, 1-year, and 2-year survival rates were of 69.5%, 31.8%, and 4.1% (mean 233 days), respectively. Results depended significantly on the number of metastases, stage, time of treatment, and use of oral chemotherapy. Ascites, jaundice, percentage of hepatic replacement, and treatment protocol also had some influence. Sex, age, primary site, elevation of tumor markers, presence of other metastatic lesions, portal vein involvement, and difference in type of chemotherapy had no prognostic significance [62]. The drugs most frequently in use are cisplatin, mitomycin C and doxorubicin. Encouraging results associated with minimal side effects were observed in a series of 61 patients treated by chemoembolization with an doxorubicin/mitomycin C Lipiodol suspension, as the 1-year survival rate estimated by the Kaplan-Meier method was 43% and the median

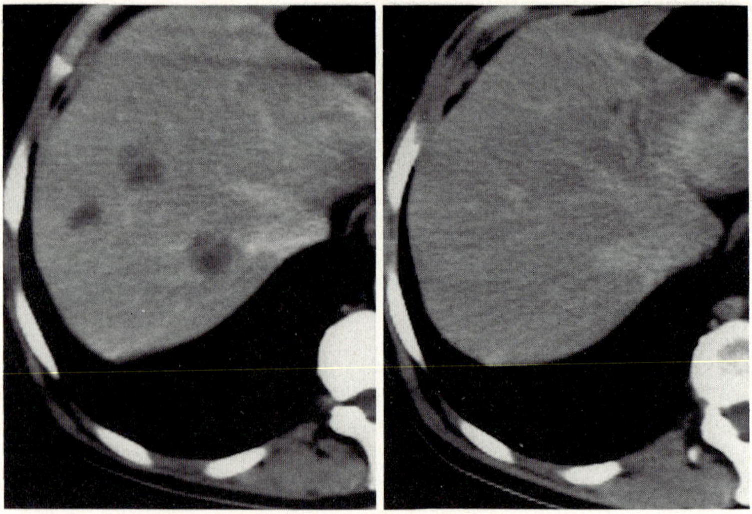

Fig. 8.8. Patient with metastases of colorectal cancer. Patient had three courses of chemoembolization using 15 mg mitomycin C, 1000 mg 5-FU, and 6 ml Lipiodol after embolization with 1 g Ivalon (250–500 μm). *Left*, before treatment; *right*, 15 months later

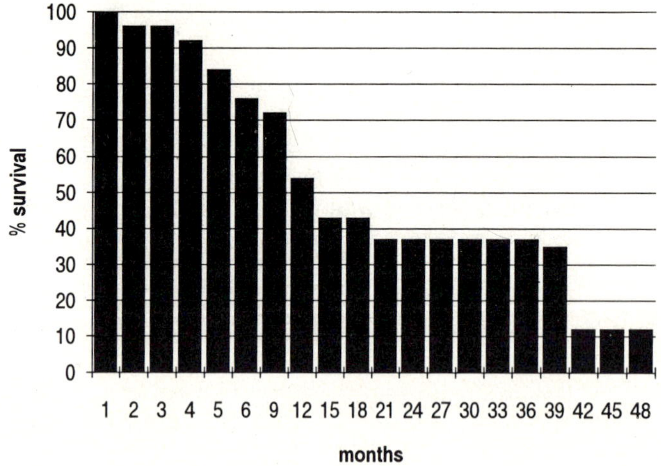

Fig. 8.9. Actuarial survival of patients treated by chemoembolization for metastatic liver disease in Cantonal Hospital of Fribourg (21 colorectal, 6 others)

survival time 337 days [63]. Survival of patients with liver metastases of various origin treated by chemoembolization at our institution is shown in Fig. 8.9.

Controlled randomized studies comparing the efficiency of chemoembolization versus standard infusion therapy are still lacking. Little is known about

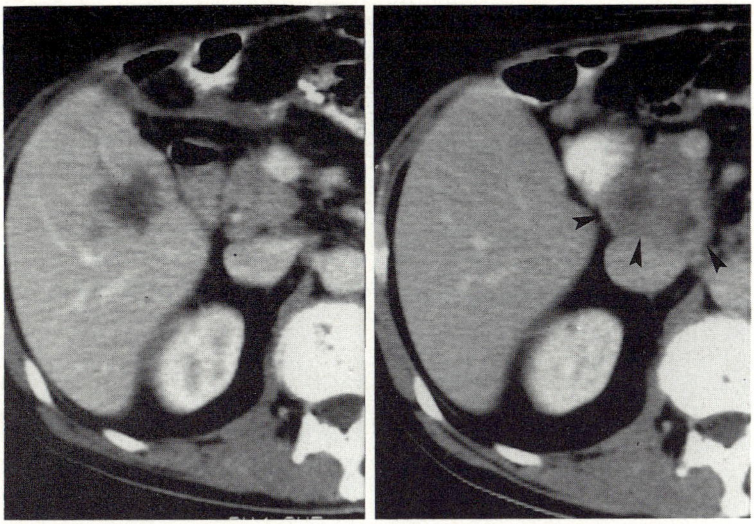

Fig. 8.10. Patient with metastases of colorectal cancer. *Left*, before treatment; *Right*, 1 year after treatment. There is no more tumor seen in the liver, but gross peripancreatic adenopathy appears (*arrowheads*). Retrospectively, small opacity which was misinterpreted as being a part of duodenum might have corresponded to a small lymph node metastasis photos.

the correct choice of chemotherapeutic agents and the correct way to combine these with embolization. Recurrences in form of distant metastases (Fig. 8.10) call for some sort of systemic therapy, the type of which is still to be found.

8.4 Complications and Side Effects of Regional Chemotherapy

Complications occurring after chemoembolization may be induced by the drug, embolization, pump or catheter, or contrast medium.

Mortality after chemoembolization is often related to hemorrhage of the tumor, liver failure [64], or septicemia [65]. Liver failure after chemoembolization is mostly encountered in the group of cirrhotic patients with hepatocellular carcinomas and is rarely found in patients treated for metastases. As cirrhotic parenchyma depends on a much higher proportion of perfusion from arterial blood than normal liver parenchyma, it is more affected by embolization and prone to end in liver failure. However, liver failure belongs to the natural history of the disease as is also a frequent cause of death of untreated patients.

Portal blood carries intestinal germs normally destroyed by liver macrophages. However, when they reach necrotic liver or tumor tissue they find a favorable field for growth. This mechanism is probably the main cause of infection (Fig. 8.11) encountered after chemoembolization. Before chemoembolization, we

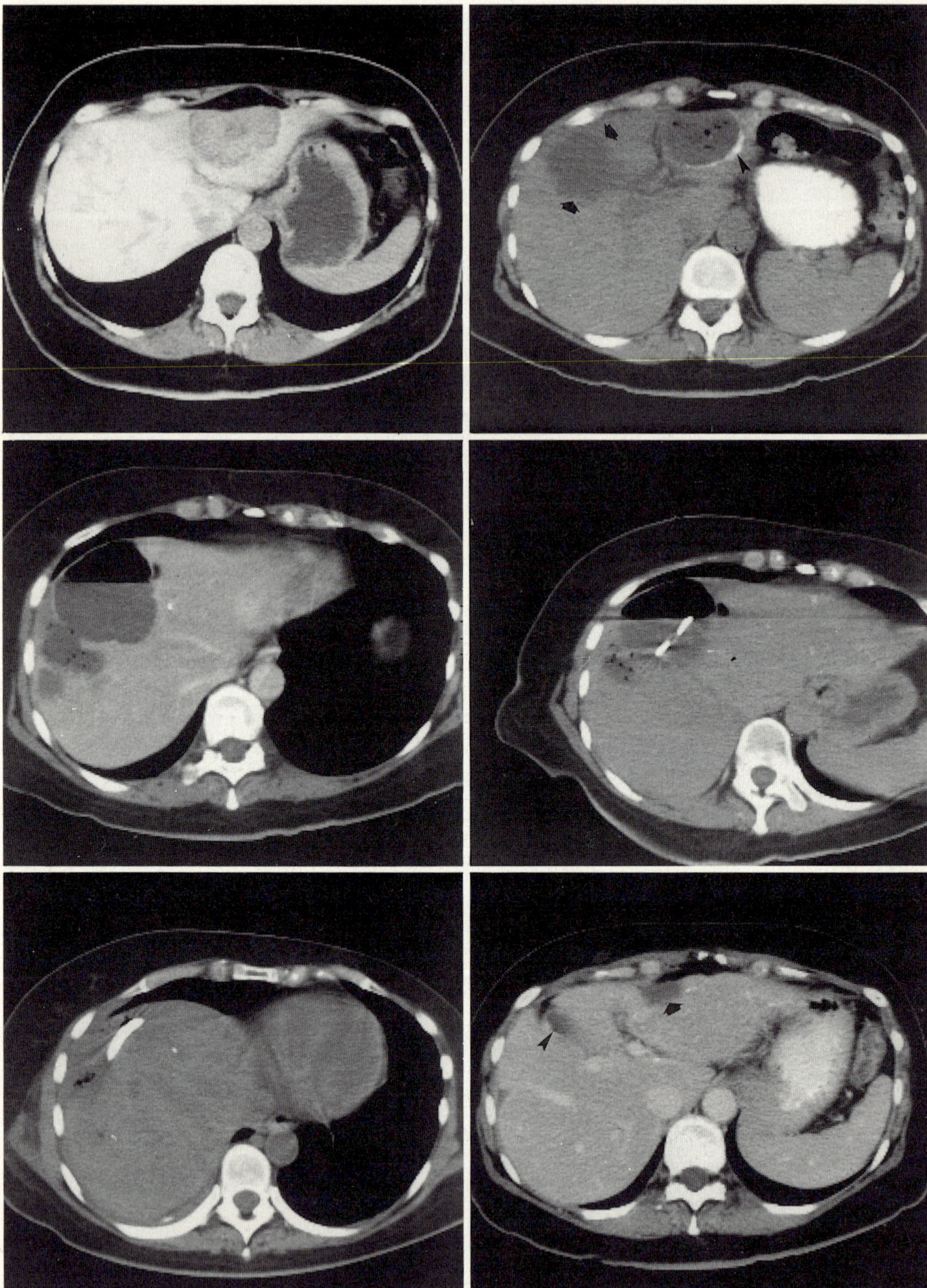
a
b
c
d
e
f

prepare the colon as for a colonic operation. Two cleaning enemas are performed the day before and on the day of the procedure. Antiobiotic prophylaxis with intravenous ceftriaxone is given before, during, and 1 day after the procedure. With this protocol we have never experienced infection.

Because of recirculation, drug-induced systemic complications or side effects are also encountered in regional chemotherapy. They are less marked or less frequent because of a lower concentration of the drug in systemic circulation. Complications or side effects depend on the type and quantity of the injected drug.

Besides tumor necrosis, regional chemotherapy induces alterations in liver parenchyma. Toxic damage such as necroses of single cells or groups of cells and cholestasis are found in about one-third of cases. After chemoembolization the effects are more marked than with perfusion alone, and necrosis of liver tissue, arteries, and bile ducts may be found. Elevation of serum bilirubin not attributable to tumor progression is related to so-called chemical hepatitis. The major complication encountered is sclerosing cholangitis [66], which is related to intraarterial perfusion with 5-FU and FUDR and occurs in about 15% of patients. Sclerosing cholangitis (Fig. 8.12) is generally encountered in the group of patients treated for liver metastasis of colorectal carcinomas as these are the drugs frequently used. Besides the toxic effect of 5-FU and FUDR, ischemic mechanisms are postulated [67]. Doxorubicin, mitomycin, or cisplatin do not appear to have the same potentiality in inducing sclerosing cholangitis. Sclerosing cholangitis should be suspected in the presence of unexplained elevation of alkaline phosphatase and bilirubin, and chemotherapy should then be suspended [68].

Gastroduodenal ulcers and gastritis are known complications of regional chemotherapy [69]. They are related to the toxic effects on the mucosa due to reflux of chemotherapeutic drugs in arteries feeding the stomach and the duodenum (the gastric arteries and the gastroduodenal artery). This type of complication is less prone to occur with chemoembolization as the mixture of Lipiodol and drugs can be delivered in a superselective controlled manner.

Seldom, infarction of portions of the liver occurs, despite the dual blood supply to the liver. It occurs not only in cirrhotic patients but also in patients with noncirrhotic liver parenchyma and normal portal circulation.

Fig. 8.11a–f. Infarction and abscess formation in patient with liver metastasis of breast cancer who refused resection. **a** Immediately after chemoembolization. Note hyperdensity of liver and tumor. **b** One week later. Note extensive necrosis of tumor with gas formation. Hyperdense rim (*arrowhead*) corresponds to Lipiodol accumulation. Note appearance of hypodensity in liver parenchyma (*arrows*). **c** Two weeks after beginning of treatment. Hypodense infarcted lesion transformed into abscess with gas formation. **d** Percutaneous placement under CT guidance of a drainage catheter. **e** Three weeks after beginning of treatment. Collapse of abscess cavity. Catheter still in place. **f** One year later. Biopsy-confirmed cystic degeneration of metastasis (*arrow*). Small scar related to abscess can still be seen (*arrowhead*)

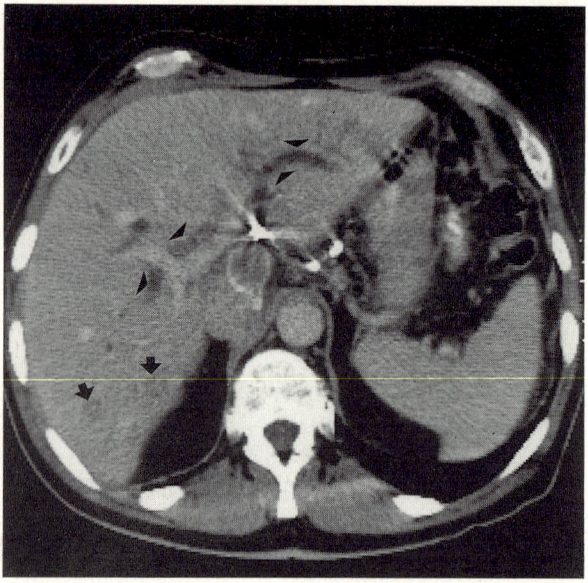

Fig. 8.12. Sclerosing cholangitis. One year after beginning of treatment of patient with multiple metastases of colorectal cancer (*small arrows*). Note dilatation of biliary ducts (*arrowheads*) Metallic artifacts are produced by coils used for "vascular remodeling." Patient was treated by a biliary stent and died 3 months later

Ischemic cholecystitis and gallbladder infarction have also been found and are related to embolization of particulate material in the cystic artery [70]. Prophylactic cholecystectomy, although discussed, does not seem to be necessary. Because of delayed gallstone formation, cholecystectomy has been recommended in patients receiving intraarterial chemotherapy before hepatectomy [71].

Compared to surgically implanted catheters, those placed in the hepatic artery using the transfemoral route (the radiological approach) tend to induce fewer complications, as they remain in place for a few hours to a few days only and are immediately withdrawn afterwards. Thrombosis of the hepatic artery is found in up to 35% of the patients with surgically placed catheters whereas this complication is only anecdotally described with catheters placed radiologically. Perforation of viscera is generally found with surgically placed catheters. Local complications due to catheters placed surgically using the left radial approach are frequent. Ischemia of the forearm and disappearance of the radial pulse necessitating the interruption of chemotherapy are found in a significant number of patients [72]. Hematoma in the groin is the complication found most frequently when using the transfemoral approach; these hematomas generally need no treatment.

Complications related to the pump pocket are infections and skin erosions. Pump failures occur rarely and are most often seen with early models.

Like all procedures used in radiology, there is a small but definite risk of contrast medium related complication. The usual precautions concerning allergy and heart- or renal-related pathology must be taken. Estimated mortality related to modern low-osmolarity contrast media is about one in 200000 patients. Severe complications such as heart failure or lung edema occur in about one in 3000 patients.

References

1. Sigurdson ER, Ridge JA, Kemeny N, Daly JM (1987) Tumor and liver drug uptake following hepatic artery and portal vein infusion. J Clin Oncol 5: 1836–1840
2. Collins JM (1984) Pharmacologic rationale for regional drug delivery. J Clin Oncol 2: 498–504
3. Collins JM (1986) Pharmacologic rationale for hepatic arterial therapy. In: Herfarth C, Schlag P, Hohenberger P (eds) Therapeutic strategies in primary and metastatic liver cancer. Springer, Berlin Heidelberg New York, pp 140–148. (Recent results in cancer research, vol 100)
4. Collins JM (1986) Pharmacologic rationale for hepatic arterial therapy. In Herfarth C, Schlag P, Hohenberger P (eds) Therapeutic strategies in primary and metastatic liver cancer. Springer, Berlin Heidelberg New York, p 143 (Recent results in cancer Research vol 100)
5. Michels NA (1955) Blood supply and anatomy of the upper abdominal organs. Lippincott, Philadelphia, pp 152–154, 256–259, 374–375
6. Cho KJ, Andrews JC, Williams DM, Doenz F, Guy GE (1989) Hepatic arterial chemotherapy: role of angiography. Radiology 173: 783–791
7. Chuang VP, Wallace S (1980) Hepatic arterial redistribution for intraarterial infusion of hepatic neoplasms. Radiology 135: 295–299
8. Sone Y, Arai Y, Tohyama N, Kido C (1991) Effect of posture for drug distribution in hepatic arterial infusion chemotherapy. 5th International Conference on Advances in Regional Cancer Treatment, June 17–19, Rosenheim
9. Miller DL, Carrasquillo JA, Lutz RJ, Chang AE (1989) Hepatic perfusion during hepatic artery infusion chemotherapy: evaluation with perfusion CT and perfusion scintigraphy. J Comput Assist Tomogr 13(6): 958–964
10. Andrews JC, Williams DM, Shapiro B, Ensminger WD (1989) Low infusion rate digital subtraction angiography to predict regional perfusion in hepatic arterial chemotherapy. Cardiovasc Intervent Radiol 12(5): 277–280
11. Lefor AT, Hughes KS, Shiloni E, Steinberg SM, Vetto JT, Papa MZ, Sugarbaker PH, Chang AE (1988) Intra-abdominal extrahepatic disease in patients with colorectal hepatic metastases. Dis Colon Rectum 31: 100–103
12. Pettavel J (1988) Intra-arterial chemotherapy using a pump. Antibiot Chemother 40: 36–40
13. Aeberhard P (1988) Intra-arterial chemotherapy without pump. Antibio Chemother 40: 41–50
14. Martin JK Jr, O'Connell MJ, Wieand HS, Fitzgibbons RJ Jr, Mailliard JA, Rubin J, Nagorney DM, Tschetter LK, Krook JE (1990) Intra-arterial floxuridine vs systemic fluorouracil for hepatic metastases from colorectal cancer. A randomized trial. Arch Surg 125: 1022–1027
15. Daly JM, Kemeny N, Sigurdson E, Oderman P, Thom A (1987) Regional infusion for colorectal hepatic metastases. A randomized trial comparing the hepatic artery with the portal vein. Arch Surg 122: 1273–1277
16. Fisher ER, Turnbull TR (1955) The cytological demonstration and significance of tumor cells in the mesenteric venous blood in patients with colorectal cancer. Surg Gynecol Obstet 100: 102–106
17. Wiggers T, Jeekel J, Arends JW, Brinkhorst AP, Kluck HM et al. (1988) No-touch isolation technique in colon cancer: a controlled prospective trial. Br J Surg 75: 409–415

18. Taylor I, Rowling JT, West C (1979) Adjuvant cytotoxic liver perfusion for colorectal cancer. Br J Surg 66: 833–837
19. Beart RW Jr, Moertel CG, Wieand HS, Leigh JE, Windschitl HE, van Heerden JA, Fitzgibbons RJ Jr, Wolff BG (1990) Adjuvant therapy for resectable colorectal carcinoma with fluorouracil administered by portal vein infusion. A study of the Mayo Clinic and the North Central Cancer Treatment Group. Arch Surg 125(7): 897–901
20. Metzger U, Laffer U, Aeberhard P, Arigoni M, Arma S, Barras J, Egli R, Martinoli S, Mueller W, Schweizer W (1990) Randomized multicenter trial of adjuvant intraportal chemotherapy for colorectal cancer SAKK 40/81: an interim report. Acta Chir Scand 156: 467–474
21. Wereldsma JC, Bruggink ED, Meijer WS, Roukema JA, van Putten WL (1990) Adjuvant portal liver infusion in colorectal cancer with 5-fluorouracil/heparin versus urokinase versus control. Results of a prospective randomized clinical trial (colorectal adenocarcinoma trial I). Cancer 65(3): 425–432
22. O'Connell MJ (1990) Is portal-vein fluorouracil hepatic infusion effective colon cancer surgical adjuvant therapy? (Editorial) J Clin Oncol 8: 1454–1456
23. Metzger U (1990) Adjuvante Therapie des Kolonkarzinoms. Schweiz Med Wochenschr 120: 1149–1158
24. Moertel CG, Fleming TR, Mcdonald JS, Haller DG, Lautie JA et al. (1990) Levamisole and fluorouracil for adjuvant chemotherapy of resected carcinoma. N Engl J Med 322: 352–358
25. Cunliffe WJ, Sugarbaker PH (1989) Gastrointestinal malignancy: rationale for adjuvant therapy using early postoperative intraperitoneal chemotherapy. Br J Surg 76: 1082–1090
26. Sugarbaker PH, Gianola FJ, Speyer JC, Wesley R, Barofsky I, Meyers CE (1985) Prospective, randomized trial of intravenous versus intraperitoneal 5-fluorouracil in patients with advanced primary colon or rectal cancer. Surgery 98: 414–422
27. August DA, Sugarbaker PH, Ottow RT, FJ, Schneider PD (1985) Hepatic resection of colorectal metastases. Influence of clinical factors and adjuvant intraperitoneal 5-fluorouracil via Tenckhoff catheter on survival. Ann Surg 201: 210–218
28. Sugarbaker PH, Graves T, DeBruijn EA, Cunliffe WJ, Mullins RE, Hull WE, Oliff L, Schlag P (1990) Early postoperative intraperitoneal chemotherapy as an adjuvant therapy to surgery for peritoneal carcinomatosis from gastrointestinal cancer: pharmacological studies. Cancer Res 50: 5790–5794
29. Mavligit GM, Zukiwski AA, Charnsangavej C, Carrasco CH, Wallace S, Gutterman JU (1992) Regional biologic therapy. Hepatic arterial infusion of recombinant human tumor necrosis factor in patients with liver metastases. Cancer 69: 557–561
30. Park C, Choi SI, Kim H, Yoo HS, Lee YB (1990) Distribution of Lipiodol in hepatocellular carcinoma. Liver 10(2): 72–78
31. Katagiri Y, Mabuchi K, Itakura T, Naora K, Iwamoto K, Nozu Y, Hirai S, Ikeda N, Kawai T (1989) Adriamycin-Lipiodol suspension for i.a. chemotherapy of hepatocellular carcinoma. Cancer Chemother Pharmacol 23(4): 238–242
32. Okazaki M, Higashihara H, Koganemaru F, Nakamura T, Kitsuki H, Hoaschi T, Makuuchi M (1991) Intraperitoneal hemorrhage from hepatocellular carcinoma: emergency chemoembolization or embolization. Radiology 180: 647–651
33. Audisio RA, Doci R, Mazzaferro V, Bellegotti L, Tommasini M, Montalto F, Marchiano A, Piva A, DeFazio C, Damascelli B et al. (1990) Hepatic arterial embolization with microencapsulated mitomycin C for unresectable hepatocellular carcinoma in cirrhosis. Cancer 66(2): 228–236
34. Mantravadi RVP, Spigos DG, Tan WS, Felix EL (1982) Intraarterial yttrium 90 in the treatment of hepatic malignancy. Radiology 142: 783–786
35. Nakao N, Ishikura R, Miura K, Takahashi H, Miura T (1987) Transcatheter arterial embolization in hepatoma complicated with obstructive jaundice. Cardiovasc Intervent Radiol 10: 40–42
36. Shibata T, Sasaki Y, Imaoka S, Nagano H, Iwanaga T, Fujita M, Ishiguro S (1990) Evaluation of preoperative chemoembolization using ethiodized oil, cisplatin and gelatin sponge (sandwich therapy) for hepatocellular carcinoma. Nippon Geka Gakkai Zasshi 91(7): 859–863

37. Fujio N, Sakai K, Kinoshita H, Hirohashi K, Kubo S, Iwasa R, Lee KC (1989) Results of treatment of patients with hepatocellular carcinoma with severe cirrhosis of the liver. World J Surg 13(2): 211–217
38. Sasaki Y, Imaoka S, Kasugai H, Fujita M, Kawamoto S, Ishiguro S, Kojima J, Ishikawa O, Ohigashi H, Furukawa H et al. (1987) A new approach to chemoembolization therapy for hepatoma using ethiodized oil, cisplatin, and gelatin sponge. Cancer 60(6): 1194–1203
39. Castrucci M, Sironi S, Vanzulli A, Angeli E, Venturini M, Mellone R, Taccagni G, Cantaboni A, Marenghi C, Ferrari G et al. (1990) Valutazione istologica postoperatoria dell'epatocarcinoma trattato mediante chemioembolizzazione. Radiol Med (Torino) 80(1–2): 79–84
40. Nagasue N, Galizia G, Kohno H, Chang YC, Hayashi T, Yamanoi A, Nakamura T, Yukaya H (1989) Adverse effects of preoperative hepatic artery chemoembolization for resectable hepatocellular carcinoma: a retrospective comparison of 138 liver resections. Surgery 106(1): 81–86
41. Hwang TL, Chen MF, Lee TY, Chen TJ, Lin DY, Liaw YF (1987) Resection of hepatocellular carcinoma after transcatheter arterial embolization. Reevaluation of the advantages and disadvantages of preoperative embolization. Arch Surg 122: 756–759
42. Falkson G, Cnaan A, Schutt AJ, Ryan LM, Falkson HC (1988) TI prognostic factors for survival in hepatocellular carcinoma. Cancer Res 48: 7314–7318
43. Attali P, Prod'Homme S, Pelletier G et al. (1987) Prognostic factors in patients with hepatocellular carcinoma. Attempts for the selection of patients with prolonged survival. Cancer 59: 2108–2111
44. Okuda K, Ohtsuki T, Obata H, Tomimatsu M, Okazaki N, Hasegawa H, Nakajima Y, Ohnishi K (1985) Natural history of hepatocellular carcinoma and prognosis in relation to treatment. Study of 850 patients. Cancer 56: 918–928
45. Sato Y, Fujiwara K, Ogata I, Ohta Y, Hayashi S, Oka Y, Furui S, Oka H (1985) Transcatheter arterial embolization for hepatocellular carcinoma. Benefits and limitations for unresectable cases with liver cirrhosis evaluated by comparison with other conservative treatments. Cancer 55: 2822–2825
46. Pelletier G, Roche A, Ink O, Anciaux ML, Derhy S, Rougier P, Lenoir C, Attali P, Etienne JP (1990) A randomized trial of hepatic arterial chemoembolization in patients with unresectable hepatocellular carcinoma. J Hepatol 11: 181–184
47. Ohnishi K, Tanabe Y, Ryu M, Isono K, Yamamoto Y, Usui S, Hiyama Y, Goto N, Iwama S, Sugita S et al. (1987) Prognosis of hepatocellular carcinoma smaller than 5 cm in relation to treatment: study of 100 patients. Hepatology 7: 1285–1290
48. Musset D, Gorce F, Roche A (1985) Embolisation des métastases hépatiques. Ann Gastroenterol Hepatol (Paris) 162: 849–859
49. Roche A, Franco D, Dhumeaux D, Bismuth H (1979) Emergency hepatic arterial embolization for secondary hypercalcemia in hepatocellular carcinoma. Radiology 133: 315–316
50. Sato Y, Fujiwara K, Furui S, Ogata I, Oka Y, Hayashi S, Ohta Y, Iio M, Oka H (1985) Benefit of transcatheter arterial embolization for ruptured hepatocellular carcinoma complicating liver cirrhosis. Gastroenterology 89: 157–159
51. Nouchi T, Nishimura M, Maeda M, Funatsu T, Hasumura Y, Takeuchi J (1984) Transcatheter arterial embolization of ruptured hepatocellular carcinoma associated with liver cirrhosis. Dig Dis Sci 29: 1137–1141
52. Hsu HC, Wei TC, Tsang YM, Wu MZ, Lin YH, Chuang SM (1986) Histologic assessment of resected hepatocellular carcinoma after transcatheter hepatic arterial embolization. Cancer 57: 1184–1191
53. Sitzman JV, Order SE, Klein JL et al. (1987) Conversion by new treatment modalities of nonresectable to resectable hepatocellular cancer. J Clin Oncol 5: 1566
54. Roche A (1991) Indication, contre-indications, résultats des chimio-embolisations. Les questions du chirurgien, les réponses du radiologue en pathologie hépatique et pancréatique. 45èmes Journées du service de Radiologie, Hôpital St-Antoine,
55. Miyayama S, Matsui O, Kameyama T, Hirose J, Konishi H, Chyotoh S, Kadoya M, Takashima T (1990) Angiographic anatomy of arterial branches to the caudate lobe of the liver with special

reference to its effect on transarterial embolization of hepatocellular carcinoma. Rinsho Hoshasen 35(3): 353–359

56. Wakasa K, Sakurai M, Kuroda C, Marukawa T, Monden M, Okamura J, Kurata A (1990) Effect of transcatheter arterial embolization on the boundary architecture of hepatocellular carcinoma. Cancer 65: 913–919
57. Kato T, Niwa M, Saito Y, Ogoshi K, Shimizu K, Nashimoto A, Kato K, Akai S (1990) Evaluation of quality of life in arterial infusion chemotherapy of hepatocellular carcinoma. Gan To Kagaku Ryoho 17(8 Pt 2): 1623–1628
58. Marlink RG, Lokich JJ, Robins JR, Clouse ME (1990) Hepatic arterial embolization for metastatic hormone-secreting tumors. Technique, effectiveness, and complications. Cancer 65(10): 2227–2232
59. Odurny A, Birch SJ (1985) Hepatic arterial embolisation in patients with metastatic carcinoid tumours. Clin Radiol 36: 597–602
60. Stockmann F, von Romatowski HJ, Reimold WV, Schuster R, Creutzfeldt W (1984) Hepatic artery embolization for treatment of endocrine gastrointestinal tumors with liver metastases. Z Gastroenterol 22: 652–660
61. Sasaki Y, Imaoka S, Masutani S, Nagano H, Ohashi I, Kameyama M, Fukuda I, Ishikawa O, Ohigashi H, Hiratsuka M et al. (1990) Chemoembolization for liver metastasis from colorectal cancer. Gan To Kagaku Ryoho 17(8): 1661–1664
62. Yamashita Y, Takahashi M, Koga Y, Saito R, Nanakawa S, Hatanaka Y, Sato N, Nakashima K, Urata J, Yoshizumi K et al. (1990) Prognostic factors in liver metastases after transcatheter arterial embolization or arterial infusion. Acta Radiol 31(3): 269–274
63. Inoue H, Kobayashi H, Itoh Y, Shinohara S (1989) Treatment of liver metastases by arterial injection of Adriamycin/mitomycin C lipiodol suspension. Acta Radiol 30: 603–608
64. Venook AP, Stagg RJ, Lewis BJ, Chase JL, Ring EJ, Maroney TP, Hohn DC (1990) Chemoembolization for hepatocellular carcinoma. J Clin Oncol 8(6): 1108–1114
65. Allison DJ, Jordan H, Hennessy O (1985) Therapeutic embolisation of the hepatic artery: a review of 75 procedures. Lancet 1(8429): 595–599
66. Herrmann G, Lorenz M, Kirkowa-Reimann M, Hottenrott C, Hubner K (1987) Morphological changes after intra-arterial chemotherapy of the liver. Hepatogastroenterology 34(1): 5–9
67. Ludwig J, Kim CH, Wiesner RH, Krom RA (1989) Floxuridine-induced sclerosing cholangitis: an ischemic cholangiopathy? Hepatology 9(2): 215–218
68. Fukuzumi S, Moriya Y, Makuuchi M, Terui S (1990) Serious chemical sclerosing cholangitis associated with hepatic arterial 5FU and MMC chemotherapy. Eur J Surg Oncol 16(3): 251–255
69. Chuang VP, Wallace S, Stroehlein J, Yap HY, Patt YZ (1981) Hepatic artery infusion chemotherapy: gastroduodenal complications. AJR Am J Roentgenol 137: 347–350
70. Takayasu K, Moriyama N, Muramatsu Y, Shima Y, Ushio K, Yamada T, Kishi K, Hasegawa H (1985) Gallbladder infarction after hepatic artery embolization. AJR Am J Roentgenol 144: 135–138
71. Jeng KS, Chiang HJ (1989) Delayed formation of gallstone after transcatheter arterial embolization for hepatocellular carcinoma. Is elective cholecystectomy advisable during hepatectomy? Arch Surg 124(11): P1319–P1322
72. Moran KT, Halpin DP, Zide RS, Oberfield RA, Jewell ER (1988) Long-term brachial artery catheterization: ischemic complications. J Vasc Surg 8(1): 76–78

Subject Index

α-fetoprotein 20
Anatomy of the liver 1
  biliary ducts 5
  caudate lobe 3
  hepatic arteries 5
  hepatic arteries variation 6
  hepatic veins 2
  lymphatic drainage 5
  portal vein 4
  variation of hepatic arterial supply 6
Angiography 28
  catheters 28
  combination with other imaging modalities 25, 26, 28
  digital subtraction 28, 29
  splenoportography 29, 30
  superselective 28
  transhepatic portography 30
Angiosarcoma 14
Arterial Ligature, see Dearterialization
Arteries, see also hepatic arteries
  coil occlusion of 81
  flow pattern in 83
  remodeling of 81, 82

Biliary ducts 5
  invasion of 12, 18
Biochemical tests 19, 20
Biopsy, percutaneous of liver 34–39
  complications 38, 39
  hemangioma 38
  malignant lesions 35–38
Blood supply to the liver 23
Budd-Chiari Syndrome 30

Calcifications in liver tumors 21, 23
Caudate lobe 3
CEA 20
Chemoembolization, see also Embolization 93–105
  complications and side effects of 101–105
  contraindications 93–95
  cystic necrosis of tumors after 96
  hepatocellular carcinoma and 97–99
  indications 93–94
  liver metastases of neuroendocrine tumors and 99
  liver metastases of non-neuroendocrine tumors and 99–101
  protocols used in 94
Chemotherapy, regional 79
  adjuvant intraperitoneal 87
  adjuvant intraportal 86
  chemoembolization, see Chemoembolization
  complications and side effects of 101–105
  intraarterial perfusion 85, 86, 88
  pharmacodynamics and 79–81
  portal versus intraarterial 86
  radiological way 88–101
  surgical way 84–88
  vascular remodeling 81
Chemotherapy, systemic 74
  drugs used 74, 75
  hepatocellular carcinoma 75, 76
  liver metastases 76, 77
  response to 74–77
Child and Turcotte classification 46
Cholangiocarcinoma 14, 27, 33
  Caroli's disease 14
  clonorchis sinensis infestation 14
  Klatskin tumors 14
Cholangiography, percutaneous, transhepatic 33
Clonorchis sinensis infestation 14
Computed tomography (CT) 23
  CT arteriography 25
  CT lipiodol 25, 40
  CT portography 25, 26
  delayed CT scanning 24, 25
  dynamic CT scanning 23, 24
  injection protocols 24
  spiral CT 23, 24
Cryosurgery 57

Dearterialization 55
results 56, 57
techniques 56

Embolization, see also Chemoembolization 91–93
hemorrhage control and 93
materials used for 91
Ethanol injection therapy 70
complications of 72
patient selection 70
results 72
technique 70, 71

Fatty Infiltration of liver 34
Fibrolamellar hepatocellular carcinoma 13
Fibrosarcomas 15
Flow in arteries, patterns of 83, 84

Hemangioendothelioma 14
Hemangioma
biopsy of 38, 39
scintigraphy of 31
Hepatectomy see Liver resection
Hepatic arteries, see also Arteries
anatomy 5
variations of 6
Hepatic veins 2
invasion of 12
Hepatoblastoma 14
Hepatocellular carcinoma
chemoembolization and 97
chemoembolization of 97–99
chemotherapy, see Chemotherapy systematic or Chemotherapy regional
clinical manifestation of 18, 19
computed tomography of 32
dearterialization in 51
epidemiology 9
epidemiology – relation to cirrhosis 11
epidemiology – relation to hepatitis 9, 10
epidemiology – relation to toxins 10, 11
fibrolamellar 13
hepatic resection in 50–53
metastatic spread of 13
Okuda's staging 47
pathology 12
ultrasonography of 31, 32

Kaposi sarcoma 34
Klatskin tumors 14

Lead time bias 74, 75
Leiomyosarcomas 15
Liver enzymes 19, 20
Liver resection 44
cirrhosis and 46
complications 54, 55
contraindications 46
criteria for resection 44
factors influencing survival 48
hepatectomy 48
hepatocellular carcinoma 50
localization of tumors 45
metastases of colorectal carcinoma 51–53
metastases of non colorectal neoplasms 51–54
recurrence of tumor 50
results 48, 50–51
role of imaging 44
segmentectomy 48
survival 51, 52
tumor margin, role of 45
types of 48, 49
Lymphatic drainage of the liver 5
Lymphoma 9, 34

Magnetic resonance 27
angiography 27
contrast agents 27
Markers 19, 20
α-fetoprotein 20
CEA 20
Mesenchymal tumors 14
Mesenchymomas 15
Metastases in liver 15, 16
chemoembolization for 99–101
chemotherapy, see chemotherapy systemic or chemotherapy regional
clinical manifestation of 19
computed tomography of 33
cryosurgery in 57
dearterialization for 55–57
hepatic resection for 51–53
radiotherapy, see radiotherapy
transplantation for 57
ultrasonography of 32
Metastatic inefficiency 16
Metastatic spread of hepatocellular carcinoma 13

Nuclear medicine see Scintigraphy

Okuda's staging of primary liver cancer 47

Perfusion of liver 3–5, 25, 84
Plain films 20, 21
Portal veins 4
invasion of 12, 44
Pugh's classification 47

Radiolabeled antibodies 65
Radiotherapy 62
^{131}I labeled lipiodol 65
chemotherapy and 67
complications of 63, 64
curative intension and 63
external 62
implantation of radioactive seeds 64
internal 64
palliative intension and 63
radiation hepatitis and 63
radiolabeled antibodies 65
tolerance of liver to radiation 62
yttrium-^{90} 64–66
Response rate to therapy 74
Rhabdomyosarcomas 15

Scintigraphy 30, 31
adenomas 31
focal nodular hyperplasia 31
hemangiomas 31
Seeds, radioactive, see radiotherapy
Segmentectomy see Liver resection
Splenoportography 29, 30
Staging of liver lesions 39, 40, 44

Transhepatic portography 30
Transplantation 58
contraindications to 59
indications for 58
liver neoplasms and 58

Ultrasound
cool doppler 22
conventional 21
Duplex doppler 22
intraoperative 22

Variation of hepatic arterial supply 6
Vascular remodeling, see also Chemotherapy, regional 81

Springer-Verlag and the Environment

We at Springer-Verlag firmly believe that an international science publisher has a special obligation to the environment, and our corporate policies consistently reflect this conviction.

We also expect our business partners – paper mills, printers, packaging manufacturers, etc. – to commit themselves to using environmentally friendly materials and production processes.

The paper in this book is made from low- or no-chlorine pulp and is acid free, in conformance with international standards for paper permanency.

Printing: Mercedesdruck, Berlin
Binding: Buchbinderei Lüderitz & Bauer, Berlin